Anatomy of an Awesome Medical Elective

How to plan your International Student Placement and get the most out of it!

Karin Eurell

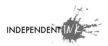

First published 2019 by Independent Ink
PO Box 1638, Carindale
Queensland 4152 Australia
independentink.com.au

Cover design by Maria Biaggini
Cover Photograph: Bijuli Timila and Bizipix | Dreamstime
Photographs: Bijuli Timila, Jon Tanner and Karin Eurell
Internal design by Independent Ink
Typeset in 11 pt Cambria by Post Pre-press Group, Brisbane

 A catalogue record for this
book is available from the
National Library of Australia

ISBN 978-0-6485547-0-7 (paperback)
ISBN 978-0-6485547-1-4 (epub)
ISBN 978-0-6485547-2-1 (kindle)

Disclaimer:
The material in this book is provided for information purposes only. The experiences discussed in this book may not necessarily be the same as the reader's experience. The reader should consult with his or her personal legal, financial and other advisors before utilising the information contained in this book. The author and the publisher assume no responsibility for any damages or losses incurred during or as a result of following this information.

Thank you to everyone who has embarked on an international student placement and provided their valuable feedback.

CONTENTS

SECTION ONE
Clarifying and Choosing Your Elective

SECTION TWO
Preparing and Doing Your Elective

SECTION THREE
Review, Reflect and Report on Your Elective Journey

FOREWORD

So why did you get into medicine?

Did it seem like a good idea at the time, or perhaps those around you said it would make an excellent career choice? Or was it more? Maybe part of your decision was based on wanting to help people?

If you do want to make a difference or want to practise medicine with only your medical knowledge and your stethoscope, then volunteering in an overseas hospital or clinic is the way to go.

But where do you start when trying to plan such a trip?

I have been asked this question often in the last 40 years of working as a GP and as a supervisor for medical students and registrars. I, too, faced the dilemma myself when I volunteered on two occasions, once in Cambodia and the second time in Tanzania. Both times I had the privilege of working with Karin Eurell, and with DocTours.

Approaching a medical elective is like anything else in medicine; it requires research.

And in terms of researching medical electives, this book is your 'go-to' text.

Karin Eurell is a professional organiser of electives. She has learnt by trial and error what is essential, and what isn't.

Anatomy of an Awesome Medical Elective guides you through each of the critical questions that must be answered for you to make the most of your overseas elective.

It starts with 'contemplation' – what to do, where to go, and how to choose between different destinations.

Next comes 'execution' – starting with the steps needed to get an appropriate elective, and then the planning phase, and lastly carrying out the elective itself.

I'm delighted Karin included Chapter 7, 'When Things Go Wrong'. Read it before you go, but make sure you re-read it when something goes wrong. I found that this usually happens some-time before the end of the first morning in your placement.

I also appreciated how much detail Karin goes into about the different issues in various countries. I've not found these issues covered as well in any other resource. If I had been given access to a book like this, I would not have felt so out of place in my volunteer placement. There are solutions to problems, if you know where to look, and this book certainly points you in the right direction of how to get help.

Make sure you also read Chapter 8, 'After Hours', about what to do with your time off. In Cambodia, it was about confronting the genocide of the past. In Tanzania, I went off to Ethiopia for the weekend. There are also many community-based options to become involved in if you have time.

Don't forget the review process at the end of your elective. What have you learnt, and what has the community gained from you being there? In their eyes, you may arrive as a medical student, but soon you will be the doctor who is relied upon for their training and expertise.

This book does not cover every challenge you will encounter, just as your medical course cannot cover every eventuality. Like your course, however, this book gives you the fundamentals you need to make the best decisions possible in the situation.

At this stage of your training, you have incredible knowledge and some skills. Learn from those around you, use your initiative, and last but not least – have the time of your life!

Thank you, Karin Eurell and DocTours, for making this incredible information available to students for their elective.

To the reader, I hope you find this information as accurate and invaluable as I have.

Dr Howard McCormick MB, BS (Hons), DRCOG, FRACGP
General Practitioner, Phillip Island, Australia
Supervisor of medical students and registrars
Chairman of Medical Education Amaco Conferences

INTRODUCTION

Your medical elective should be an experience of a lifetime!

As part of your training, you have a four to eight-week window to travel anywhere in the world and get some clinical experience in any medical field that interests you. The possibilities are endless, and so the amount of research needed may seem overwhelming. There are many choices and decisions that you need to make, such as where to go, what to do and how to organise everything.

It is certainly possible to arrange everything yourself. However, it can sometimes be difficult to track down the appropriate people, email addresses and phone numbers of who can help you coordinate your plans. Discussing and communicating your elective preferences and understanding your university's criteria for gaining credit for the elective can also be challenging, as well as contacting and getting responses from hospitals in developing countries. Gaining their commitment, reconfirming with them and convincing them that you are really coming may also be problematic. And of course, there is the fear of missing out on the opportunity and the reality of not securing the placement of your dreams.

'DocTours' has been arranging international electives for medical students for over six years. As co-founder of the company, I am passionate about travel and excel at logistics. I have visited many foreign hospitals and inspected and stayed in the local accommodation so that I can recommend the most appropriate venues for your needs. I have successfully arranged elective programs for more than 500 medical students.

With regular feedback from past travellers, I ensure that DocTours maintains up to date with information for interested students, and I use this intelligence to develop and improve what we offer. I attend and present the information I have at elective nights at many universities. And I regularly hear from past students who have travelled abroad, while also answering many of the questions of future travellers. Having travelled with groups of students on their electives to see, hear and experience everything firsthand, it has been my ultimate goal to share all of this knowledge and experience with you in this book.

You may prefer to do your elective in Australia, or in another developed country. With modern technology and communication systems, it is relatively easy to arrange somewhere (or anywhere) to go to do your elective.

However, will it be a truly life-changing and amazing experience?

Will you be talking about your adventures for the rest of your life?

Do you want to see conditions and resources that are diverse to what you normally see at home?

If the answer to these questions is 'YES', I highly recommend you look into doing your elective in any of the countries I discuss in this book. With extensive experience in Fiji, Cambodia, Nepal, Sri Lanka, Tonga and Tanzania, I will be focusing on these countries in depth.

Arranging an elective in a developing country can be time-consuming and frustrating due to limited and unreliable communication channels.

This book is not just a handy reference book; it aims to provide you with guidance in navigating the many questions you may have. So I have endeavoured to provide lots of useful information to help you choose, plan, and get the most out of your elective. You can even read about the amazing experiences enjoyed by many other students and international volunteers who have travelled before you. My goal is to take away the hassle, the stress and the confusion so that you can focus on enjoying the journey.

While this book is primarily written for Australian medical students, there is information that is useful for students from around the world, and also for medical volunteers who dream of travelling and working overseas.

As future doctors, you have the unique opportunity to explore and discover another country where you can continue to learn and develop your skills. I really want your medical elective to be rewarding, worthwhile, and an amazing experience. My philosophy is that we should all be the best at what we do.

I don't believe in taking large busloads of students into a small hospital where everyone is crowded around a patient and unable to see or hear what is going on. I like to offer a choice of attractive destinations with a variety of experiences (both during and after work), as well as safe locations, flexible arrangements, and hosts who will make you feel welcome.

You deserve to get the most out of your elective – and have the time of your life!

My goal is to help you do this.

SECTION ONE

||||||||||||||||||||||||||||||||||||||||||||||||||||||||||||||||||||||||||||||||||||||||||||||||||

Clarifying and Choosing
Your Elective

One of the most bewildering parts of doing an international elective is deciding on your country of choice and the type of experience you wish to enjoy, as the possibilities are endless.

But first things first: in this section you will gain some insight into how best to go about choosing where to do your elective, applying for your elective, and then what hoops you might need to jump through before you step on that plane and head off on an adventure of a lifetime.

With some thorough planning and organisation, and some assistance on the side, these initial steps are easy to follow and implement.

So, let's get started …

CHAPTER 1

ARRANGING AN ELECTIVE

#wheredoIstart?

Your clinical elective is an opportunity to choose an area of medicine that interests you and to spend some time experiencing life in that department. Many medical students choose to do this in their home country, such as Australia, New Zealand, Canada, the USA, or the UK; however, there are many opportunities for students to carry out their elective in a developing country.

If the idea of doing your elective in a hospital or clinic outside of your own country entices you, there are quite a number of things to consider. However, by doing some thorough research into what you need to do to make this goal a reality, the experience can run smoothly.

This chapter will focus on the criteria needed for completing an elective overseas, as well as information and inspiration that is readily available to give you a sound understanding of what you will be doing, as well as provide a good overview of what to expect when on your elective overseas.

While many medical students choose an overseas elective,

students from dentistry, nursing, and allied health are also welcomed on international placements and can gain valuable experience while putting new skills into practice.

Given that the international experience will be different, some of the main disparities between completing an elective in your home 'developed country' and abroad are also discussed.

University criteria

Each medical school has different criteria for completing electives, and so it is important to understand the requirements of your course. The major variants are:

1. What is the stage or year you require to do your elective?

    Some universities send students into the hospital system at the end of their first year, while others do so in their later or final years. Students in the earlier stages are therefore mainly observing and learning about the internal systems and processes of a hospital. Students in their later years will expect more hands-on experiences and can get more involved in working with patients under supervision of local staff.

2. The dates for your elective.

    It is ideal to understand the specific dates for your elective rotation as early as possible. You can even consider buddying up with fellow students in the same cohort with the same dates as your rotation, and then plan an overseas placement together. Some students are happy to travel solo, going where they prefer and then meeting international travellers on placement. If you choose to go with another student, apply and book well in advance to ensure that you secure the same location in your preferred areas of interest. Students often apply more than 12 months in advance for the most popular placements, and therefore I recommend that you do not delay your enquiry and application process.

3. The duration of your elective.

   With the longer placements of eight weeks, you may be able to split your attachment across two locations (e.g. four weeks domestically and the other four weeks overseas). With eight weeks (or more), why not consider travelling further afield (e.g. Africa, South America, Asia or Europe)? The longer duration gives you ample opportunity to explore the region and gain a better appreciation of the lifestyle and culture of a different tribe.

4. The major learning objectives.

   Your university may require you to choose a placement that covers a specific area of medicine, such as community medicine, emergency, health equity, or rural and remote medicine.

5. What is the university's approval process for your elective?

   Your university will need to approve your specific elective program to ensure that it meets their criteria. The criteria may include certain learning objectives so that you gain course credit for your placement. Most importantly, they will want to ensure that you have something actually lined up, and they will be interested in the safety of the destination. Therefore, the choice of country becomes important.

6. What reporting and assignments are required and when are their due dates?

Your elective is not *just* an amazing journey! You will need to complete many forms and think about your personal learning objectives. You may be required to undertake an analysis of potential risks and how you intend to manage and mitigate these risks. You are often required to report to your supervisors during your placement, and there will be a written report due at the end of your placement. Your final report may be a reflection on your observations and what you learnt about medicine, or it could be about access to medicine in a different community.

Sources of information and inspiration

Your university's Medical Society (Med Soc) may arrange an information event known as the 'electives night' during the early part of the year. On these specific nights there will be presentations from students who completed their elective the previous year, and your elective coordinator may provide details on your university's criteria and processes for undergoing your elective. There will also be presentations from organisers of elective programs, medical indemnity providers, and banks that specialise in lending to the medical profession.

These events are a valuable source of information, and they also give you the opportunity to learn more about what doing an elective entails, as well as having the opportunity to ask questions, pick up a brochure and discuss it all with your friends and peers.

If you are an Australian medical student, I also recommend that you check out the websites of the Australian Medical Student Association (AMSA), medical indemnity providers (e.g. MIPS, MDA), and the elective organisers, as there will be interesting case studies, reports and ideas on unusual placements, destinations and

activities. Some of these websites will also provide useful information about grants, funding alternatives, competitions and prizes.

Inspiration usually comes from the students who have recently
returned from their elective in a developing country. Jan, a student
from the University of New England, told me, 'I'm so thankful that
I went with DocTours, as both my placements were fantastic!
They were well organised, rewarding, and they helped me learn
so much! Thank you from the bottom of my heart for everything
that you've done. I will definitely recommend DocTours to all my
younger peers who are planning their placements at the moment.'

I am certainly delighted to hear that the students I have helped
over the years have embraced their experiences and can share
their gratification with prospective students.

Who can do their elective overseas?

Students who are studying dentistry, nursing, and allied health
are all welcome to help and learn in an international hospital or
clinic. And there is usually more opportunity to have hands-on
experience in a hospital or clinic in a developing country than gain
access to such clinical experience in Australia or other developed
countries. This is because of the limited time and resources of the
supervising doctors and the relatively large number of students
who are in training in Australia, New Zealand, Canada, the USA,
and the UK.

Hospitals in developing countries usually charge a fee for hosting
students, and this is an important revenue source for the hospital,
which they use towards paying staff and purchasing medical
supplies. So international students are appreciated. Therefore, if
you are interested in gaining more clinical experience and have the
opportunity to explore an interesting international destination,
the elective arrangers are eager to organise all of this for you.

Some locations (such as Nepal) will be happy to host students
at all stages of their training and experience. You can even choose

your dates and your duration. Your program is often flexible enough so that you can spend part of your time in a hospital, as well as do some health-related volunteer work to help the local community. This will depend on your level of training and experience (e.g. a first aid certificate or other relevant training), and you can put these skills into practice with mini-health checks, teaching the local community about first aid, health and hygiene, or even by helping the local people improve their English.

People in developing countries are often keen to learn and practise their English because it provides them with more career opportunities in tourism, hospitality, and university studies. Therefore, they are very grateful for any assistance in improving their English skills.

This is a great way to spend a few weeks of your semester break. You will learn about performing medicine in a low-resource setting, and also have the chance to practise your medical skills, explore a new country, volunteer and help others, meet new people, jazz up your CV, and have an incredible time as well!

Overview of an elective and your program

You should expect to be based in a functioning hospital (or clinic) that is staffed with local doctors, nurses, and possibly some expat staff. It could be busy with long queues of patients waiting quietly to be seen by a doctor. And it may seem inefficient due to a lack of basic diagnostic equipment and technology, or their processes may not seem to make sense. The pace might be faster, or slower than what you are used to in your home country.

You will be allocated to a supervisor (or a few supervisors) and work among a team of staff. It is suggested that you spend the first few days observing the processes, learning about typical conditions, discovering what resources are available and watching how the doctors interact with patients. Examine the medical files (they are usually in English), and ask questions when appropriate to do so. You should demonstrate that you are interested and keen to learn, and that you want to be involved and are happy to assist the staff.

Overview of an organised program

If you are thinking about joining an 'organised program', you might be wondering what exactly is arranged for you. The arranger will identify, locate, liaise, negotiate and communicate with hospitals in developing countries on your behalf. The arranger will book the best placement for you (and your family and friends), arrange airport transfers, accommodation and registration. This saves you considerable time so that you can focus on your studies. Payments for all of these services will be made in advance so you don't need to bother with the foreign exchange matters or carry large sums of cash with you overseas.

On an organised program, you will be provided with information and checklists to help you prepare for your journey. You will also be informed about what it costs to live and work in the destination. Just check on what is included in your package and what is excluded so you can budget accordingly. You can also expect to feel supported and have someone checking in on a regular basis to ensure that everything is okay. This support is certainly something that is appreciated by students and volunteers who are travelling alone and/or in a foreign environment.

I find that many students appreciate the prompt communication prior to their trip, as well as the support offered by these providers. They also find it extremely handy having someone handle the finer details of organising accommodation, airport transfers and a placement at the hospital.

One student reported that it was really nice having someone else do all the logistics. She appreciated the responsiveness, and having questions answered quickly helped to make it a great experience.

What you will learn

Your elective is an opportunity to put some of the skills that you have learnt from textbooks and at medical school into practice. It is therefore wise to be prepared to do basic tasks such as taking patient histories, undertaking examinations and observations, and learning how to scrub-in to the operating room and other relevant protocols.

Many students want to experience how other medical practitioners do things in other less-developed countries, and to help out wherever they can. During the relatively short time that you are visiting a foreign country, you should not expect to change the world. You should simply aim to learn as much as you can and try to improve people's lives – one at a time. Perhaps you could even return to the hospital again in the future as a qualified, experienced practitioner and make even more of an impact.

Disparities between 'developed' countries and 'developing' countries

You will notice many differences between hospitals and clinics in developed countries, such as Australia, New Zealand, Canada, the USA and the UK, and hospitals and clinics in developing countries. For example, access to basic diagnostic tests may be unavailable or unaffordable in a developing country, or the doctors' bedside manners may be different, their patient interactions unusual, and their approach to hand hygiene or infection control unfamiliar.

There is a lot less emphasis on hand hygiene in hospitals in less-developed countries, and the use of sterile equipment is not always possible. There can also be a shortage of gloves, and many hospital departments do not have adequate facilities for staff to even wash their hands.

Many patients can present with more advanced symptoms than you would normally see in developed countries. The available treatments could also be more limited than what you are used to.

Patients also often have to pay for their medications, syringes and needles, IV fluids and administration sets, as well as the cost of surgeries and treatments, and other dressing materials that are needed during their hospital stay. There is generally limited support from the government in developing countries for medical care, and many people can't afford private health insurance. A visit to the hospital may consume their savings; an operation and medication might be unaffordable. In some cases, if a patient and their caregiver do not go to work, it could mean that their family can't afford to eat.

To give you an idea of the more particular disparities found in hospitals and clinics in developing countries, let's have a further look at three of the countries that I have experienced.

Disparities in Nepal

Many find it eye-opening to see the disparities between Nepalese health care and that which we have in Australia, especially in relation to pre-hospital care. Most patients arrive by taxi or car, even when in a critical, life-threatening state, as the ambulances are not staffed with paramedics or qualified medical personnel. Ambulances are rather just a mode of transport for the patient, but no management of the patient or their condition is provided as they travel. Therefore, many patients arrive in severe, decompensated states, and being involved in their assessment and management is a unique experience.

Patient follow-up is inconsistent in Nepal, particularly when patients need to travel from remote areas to get to a hospital. A patient could be asked to attend a follow-up in one month; however, they actually only present for their follow-up appointment after seven to eight months. This seems to be a common situation, and patients usually tend to either continue the medication for longer than they needed to or stop a medication that they were required to continue for longer.

Disparities in Fiji

In recent years, there has been a growth in 'Non-Communicable Diseases' (NCD), particularly type 2 diabetes. Many patients initially turn to 'traditional' medicine, which can delay effective treatment, leading to severe complications that can include amputations and fatalities. The outcome of this is that there are a large number of diabetes-related amputations (often three per day at the major hospitals in Fiji, where the total population is just over 900,000).

There are also a growing number of teenage pregnancies, and there is an increasing demand for midwives and nurses who specialise in paediatric, post-natal, maternal child and women's health. These professionals also run outreach programs to conduct physical examinations and immunisations during the school terms. Medical students are often invited to join these outreach programs, and it is usually one of the highlights of the students' experiences.

There has been growing awareness of the importance of healthy living in Fiji.

Women are being encouraged to grow their own vegetables and are taught healthier cooking techniques (e.g. by reducing salt and adding herbs). These women have been empowered through education, engagement, and by taking responsibility, and this seems to be quite sustainable. However, this increased awareness has not yet had a significant impact on alcohol and kava abuse, the high amount of smoking, the levels of stress, and the consumption of junk food and general lack of physical activity.

The scenic Coral Coast running between Nadi and Suva is famous for many tourist resorts, but unfortunately it experiences a large proportion of road accidents along its beautiful, winding roads.

I once attended a morning handover meeting at the local hospital and the list of cases was extremely interesting. For example, there was a drunk who wandered onto the road the previous night and had been hit by a vehicle. Another patient died when the hospital ran out of medication. The shortage of medical supplies and basic equipment (e.g. every hospital seems to need more pulse oximeters) was prevalent.

Specialists are highly valued and are in demand, including emergency department (ED) consultants, anaesthetists, radiologists, pathologists and cardiologists. The hospitals and clinics in Fiji are keen for specialists to mentor and transfer knowledge to the local staff who are eager to learn.

I have seen lots of happy, smiling children in Fiji with pearly white teeth. One of the contributing factors for this is that children up to the age of 15 receive free dental care in Fiji. In addition, Colgate generously donates a new toothbrush and toothpaste for every child every year. After that, dental care comes at a cost that many Fijians can't afford, and therefore patients ultimately present at the hospital with toothaches. The dental teams are kept busy on a daily basis just addressing the cause of pain, and most of the time, extraction is the only solution by that stage.

Fiji welcomes volunteer dentists. This provides an opportunity to offer patients free dental care to help prevent and treat conditions at an earlier stage. Any specialist skills are advantageous, and the Fijians will screen and book in relevant patients in advance. While the hospitals in Suva and Lautoka have the largest dental clinics, the greatest need is often on the more remote islands and in their outreach programs.

Disparities in Tanzania

A doctor I know who was volunteering in Tanzania was saddened by the number of maternal and foetal deaths she encountered. At this particular hospital, there was a different level of care, and the lack of monitoring resulted in a higher number of Caesareans. Her advice to medical students wishing to do their elective in

Tanzania is to be prepared to observe and learn different medical conditions and management *without* trying to change things.

Another medical student reported that having the opportunity to move throughout the hospital freely was a privilege. She was able to assist where she could and learn the different ways of the Tanzanians' culture. Patients were usually in basic beds with mosquito nets hanging from the ceiling. Their relatives would bring food for them, and it wasn't uncommon to see a thermos of soup on the bedside table. She saw young African women naked on narrow beds in maternity, labouring with no husband or other relatives to support them.

However, she noted that there was generally a calmness about the hospital. Things were done methodically, and time was not pressured. Where you might expect chaos and clamour, people were waiting quietly to be seen.

She was struck by the stoic, non-complaining nature of the people. A teenaged Masai girl with advanced heart failure following rheumatic fever sat quietly slumped in her bed with laboured breathing as staff discussed her ongoing care and her very limited options.

The medical student was intrigued as she watched brain surgery being performed on a man in his mid-20s who had fallen off a motorbike and sustained a subdural haematoma. With no fancy craniotomy tools in sight, the surgeons used a hammer and chisel to make their way through this young man's skull to locate and release the clot. The surgeon didn't seem perturbed to have blood splashing over his sandalled feet.

A few days later, the young man was seen back in the ward, sitting up in bed, smiling and delighted that his headaches had resolved.

Even in remote Australia, both patients would have been evacuated by air to a tertiary centre.

CHAPTER 2

WHAT TO EXPECT ON YOUR ELECTIVE OVERSEAS

#whattoexpect

You probably have many questions about what to expect when visiting a developing country for your elective. You might wonder why it is such a beneficial idea, or what the inside of a foreign hospital is like, as well as what technology and medical supplies are available. And, of course, you'll want to know what you'll be doing, what you can learn and what is expected from you. You may also question how you can contribute to the patients' health care or if you will just get in the way of busy staff. These are all valid questions that I will discuss in this chapter. I have also made a couple of suggestions of what *not* to do.

Why do your elective in a developing country?

So why would you decide to jump on a plane and travel to one of the poorest countries in the developing world to work in a hospital? This is probably one of the first questions you might ask yourself when trying to decide *if* you should do it.

If you love to travel and experience new countries, are eager to work outside of your comfort zone to gain some career and personal growth, and also have an adventure on the side – why wouldn't you?

Why not spend your time in a foreign location that has a rich history, unique culture and architecture, natural beauty, native animals, as well as traditional cuisine? With the opportunity and time to visit any part of the world, it would seem a shame to stay at home and work in your local hospital. Why not work and live in a more exotic location that you can explore at leisure after work and on your weekend?

Following graduation, you will be working incredibly long hours as a junior doctor and you might not find the time to embark on a big journey in the near future. As you progress through your career, time remains scarce and you could be laden with marriage, children and a mortgage.

All the more reason to travel now – while you are young and independent.

You may have a lifelong dream to travel to remote areas of Australia, for example, to support Indigenous health, or to head across the seas to enjoy the warmth and friendliness of the Fijian islands. Or perhaps trekking the Himalayas or going on a wildlife safari in Africa entices you. Whatever you desire, why not incorporate it with the development of your career and make the most of the opportunity while you can.

Another important factor in your choice might be to travel where there could be more opportunities for *hands-on experience*. Final year students who are interested in surgery and who go overseas to work in a developing country can actually scrub-in and spend their entire elective in theatre. By fostering the trust and confidence of the surgeon, students who have done just that have been able to take on more responsibility and assist in the procedures.

Other students who have been interested in obstetrics have been able to play a role in deliveries, and some students have sutured wounds in an emergency department. These situations often occur due to a shortage of staff, and therefore students (both local and foreign) can play a role in helping with large caseloads.

It is important to note, however, that you are not *expected* to undertake any procedures that you have not been trained to do, and you should only carry out these jobs under supervision of a local doctor or medical professional. The level of hands-on work will depend on a number of factors, including: the country, hospital, patient-load, local regulations, and the remoteness of the location. The more remote parts of any country often have fewer doctors and less regulatory oversight. The larger city hospitals are often better staffed, and they may have more local students based there. They also seem to be subjected to more stringent regulations.

Wherever you go, you will have the opportunity to see and learn firsthand about conditions that are less common at home. For example, polio, TB and many tropical diseases are rarely seen in developed countries, and therefore it is interesting to see cases at all stages of their development and learn about their treatment.

As I am passionate about improving access to health care for everyone – globally – I personally think that the greatest gift you can give yourself and the people in developing countries is the role you can play in helping to teach local children, teachers and families about health and hygiene, and also about the benefits of modern medicine.

Main reasons for choosing to do an elective in a developing country

I find that students grow and gain confidence during their elective program, particularly as they get more involved with the staff and patients. Other reasons for doing your elective in a developing country include:

- To share your very useful skills with the locals; teach them about new systems and techniques.
- To learn new skills (perhaps 101 uses of a rubber glove). You will be exposed to basic medicine, improvising and learning alternative ways of doing things. Work and life back home will seem 'easy' by comparison.
- To enhance your resume, fulfil university requirements or earn Continuing Professional Development (CPD) points.
- To gain the personal satisfaction of helping people who are less fortunate than yourself.
- To explore outside your comfort zone and see something beyond the usual.
- To experience personal growth by not having the support and creature comforts you have at home. To learn another language (or at least some key words so that you can communicate more effectively).
- To meet other international volunteers, share stories, and make new friends.
- To live like the locals in homestay accommodation. It may sound confronting; however, it is great fun. Become part of the family – eat, cook, and take part in their daily lives.
- To travel and work in fabulously interesting countries.
- To experience another culture.

The above points can be further demonstrated by the following example. A medical friend of mine was on a plane that was struck by lightning. This was a terrifying moment for everyone on board, and it was followed by strong turbulence. He made the decision that he had to give something back. An epiphany – maybe! Within a couple of months, he was off to Myanmar to volunteer at an eye clinic, mainly assisting with cataract surgeries.

He expressed to me that the conditions he experienced while there were an 'eye-opener' compared to the sterile clinical environment in Australia. He was totally out of his comfort zone, given the foreign language, culture and resources; however, he became more accustomed to his surroundings over time. He adapted to the daily routine and enjoyed the banter around the dinner table at night with like-minded people.

Importantly, many impoverished locals who had no vision due to severe cataracts were now able to see. They could see their family, go to work and build a better life. It was a truly life-changing experience for them (and for the him).

Doing your elective abroad provides enormous opportunities to improve your communication skills. Triage could be challenging, particularly when working through an interpreter. Expressing decisions on whether to treat or refer patients, as well as communicating management plans and instructions in a clear and concise manner – while checking that local staff have understood you fully – will provide potential for enhanced communication skills!

Working in a team environment is invaluable when there are varied backgrounds across nursing, paramedics and other medical specialties. Sharing knowledge and experience helps everyone to learn and develop a greater appreciation of other roles that facilitate better all-round care for the patients. You may be asked to present some first aid training to local teachers, which can be an interesting and rewarding experience, and it is more powerful when delivered by a multi-disciplinary team.

The ability to work with limited resources and in an environment that may not be sterile is another challenge. Developing problem-solving skills, lateral thinking and the ability to improvise with a can-do attitude is important. In Australia, for example, where health-care budgets are being cut, learning to appreciate whatever resources you have can be an advantage.

Aims and objectives of working in a developing country

Working in a low-resource setting is not optimal; however, it is an opportunity to foster initiative and greater resourcefulness. Other life-changing career and personal development aims and objectives could include:

- To gain valuable experience working in a low/middle income country and immersing yourself in a new culture.
- To become familiar with common conditions in the developing country's population, including their pathophysiology, presentation, prognosis and treatment.
- To understand how different social attitudes might influence health outcomes.
- To gain insight into working in an environment with far fewer resources than you are used to – understanding how to cope and adapt to different settings.
- To learn how to navigate a language barrier during consultations.

Learning objectives for your medical elective

Your university course may have some expectations about what you will experience during your medical elective and these may include the following:

- To experience health care in a setting removed from your usual context.
- To appreciate the differences and similarities in the availability and allocation of resources, population sizes and characteristics, systems of health care, and culture and values between home and another nation.
- To improve and apply skills in a particular discipline, including communication and history-taking, physical

examination, and assisting the treating team as needed.
- To assist in the provision of services to the local community through volunteer programs in community health or women's shelters.

What you can expect inside foreign hospitals

Developing countries rarely have access to the modern technology and latest medical equipment common in Australia, New Zealand, Canada, the USA, or the UK. In some cases, sophisticated equipment has been donated to the hospitals in developing countries by well-meaning charities and are initially put to good use. However, over time the equipment eventually breaks down. Frequently, there are no spare parts, and no one has been trained to service or repair the equipment. Therefore, equipment may stand idle.

In public hospitals, patients often have to pay to see a doctor, as well as pay for any drugs prescribed and investigations ordered. Often, the patient has insufficient funds (or laboratory facilities are unavailable) to undertake a full blood test as part of a diagnosis. Therefore, doctors in developing countries may need to rely on their own observations and experience to diagnose and treat patients. This is what I call 'practising back-to-basics medicine', and the doctors have well-developed physical exam skills. For example: doctors may use the back of their hand to gauge temperature and determine whether a patient has a fever.

Several patients might even share a bed or take their place on the floor of the corridor, and the oxygen machine could be shared by several patients at a time by joining the tubes. When struggling with the lack of tests available, a volunteer doctor is advised: 'if the results of the blood test would not change your treatment plan, then you need to proceed without it'.

Beds could be in disrepair and everything is in short supply. Patients are waiting for fresh supplies, and doctors are waiting for equipment – because of this there are often unfortunate consequences. For example, in a Fijian hospital I visited, the well-worn mattresses resulted in ulcers on the patients, and the only mobile X-ray device was broken.

One student that I spoke to needed to take a patient's blood sample and a helpful nurse handed him a latex glove. It took him a little while to figure out that he was meant to use the glove as a tourniquet because the hospital did not have any and the gloves were also in short supply. I have also seen many consumables be recycled and reused in developing countries. For example: needles in Nepal are recapped and reused (on the same patient), and staff have developed a creative technique for recapping the needle safely to avoid needle-stick injury.

However, there is more to working in a developing country's hospital than just the 'work' you will do. Living and working in a foreign country also provides time to develop an appreciation of other cultures. Sharing a coffee in the doctors' tearoom presents many opportunities to swap stories about interesting cases, life experiences and work challenges. This is where you gain a better understanding of why and how things happen in that country. Be in the moment and soak up the experience, and adopt their perspectives and pace of life. See and learn how the other half live.

While you do not need to be fluent in the local language, working internationally will necessitate learning some of the local words and medical phrases. It is fun to learn, and both patients and staff will respond favourably to any efforts that you make to speak their language. I will discuss communication in more detail later in the book.

A student in Tanzania once commented, 'The hospital is brilliant – but there is definitely an element of the language barrier. I am constantly working on my Swahili, as well as my confidence in asking for translations. However, I do get to see and do a lot, which is exactly what I'd hoped for. Now that I have been here for a week, I know most of the names of the people on the ward, which helps.'

One student in Tonga suggested, 'If you are on the brink of deciding whether or not to embark on a voluntary experience, I would encourage you to make it happen. It is not as hard as you may think, and the life and professional experience is well worth it.'

Another student described her reasons for visiting Tanzania, by saying, 'I had no clear expectations of what the experience would be like, and I certainly didn't believe that I'd make much impact in just a few short weeks, but I was keen to help in any way I could. I spent a lot of time researching different volunteer organisations and decided on DocTours, as it seemed to be well organised and flexible enough to meet my needs. Still unsure of what I was heading into, I strode through the airport doors and headed to Africa. I had an amazing experience. This was due to the combination of a fascinating location, the opportunity to see close up how a less-developed medical system actually manages to work, and the people I was fortunate enough to meet along the way.'

Benefits for the foreign hospital

A medical student can be useful in many ways. Your contribution and level of involvement as a medical student will depend on several factors, such as:

- Your level of training, skills, attitude and willingness to assist wherever needed. With more experience and more time in your volunteer role, you will be able to build trust and gain the confidence of your supervisor.
- What you would like to get out of the experience. Are you happy to observe and assist when required (e.g. take histories, do obs, assist medical professionals under supervision)? Do you want to learn and practise new skills?

Are you prepared to undertake any tasks that help nurses with patient comfort and care?
- The location of the hospital. You need to be mindful of local requirements to comply with student medical registration and visas.
- Communication is key! You may need to repeatedly offer to help staff with specific tasks that you have been trained to do. Note that you should not be expected to undertake tasks that you have not been trained to do, and you are not expected to work alone – you should be part of a team.

Some people ask if medical students place a burden on the hospital; however, I see many of the following benefits:

- You are an extra pair of hands to help out.
- You are able to share knowledge of what you have learnt and experienced (in some countries there is no Continuing Professional Development requirement for local staff).
- You are showing people in remote areas and developing countries that you care.
- You offer tangible support. Hospitals generally charge a fee to host medical elective students and often receive donations of medical supplies.
- You allow the staff to build relationships and contacts for the future. Many students are interested in returning to a developing country after they graduate so that they can contribute even more!
- The local tourism industry gets a boost.

What you will be doing

Your main role is to observe and assist the local doctors while you are there. It is important to build a good relationship with all staff and patients, and most importantly with your supervisor. If you are working with the one doctor for several weeks or more, your enthusiasm, willingness to learn, insightful questions and offering to help will hold you in good stead. As you build their confidence and trust, you should be offered more responsibility and more involvement.

Please remember, however, that if you do not feel confident or ready, or are not trained to perform certain procedures, do not feel pressured to do so. Just politely explain that you have not been trained yet. However, don't be afraid to offer to assist when appropriate.

Your elective will most likely be based in a hospital and in a department that you have chosen. Many developing countries will also do outreach work. Medical teams will pack their portable clinic and visit remote villages, homes, schools and clinics to provide health care to the community.

If you have the opportunity to join these outreach clinics, it is worthwhile doing so because you will see patients, procedures and situations that you would not see at the hospital and therefore gain greater insights into how the locals live. Some countries also offer the opportunity to visit children at local schools, disabled centres and orphanages for an afternoon or a day each week.

Your role may vary, and it could include undertaking mini-health check-ups (taking vital signs and histories) and teaching first aid, health and hygiene. Many medical students find these experiences particularly rewarding, as they have the chance to work independently and directly with the local children while practising basic medical skills.

Some students are passionate about a career in surgery or obstetrics. Therefore, they choose to spend their entire elective in theatre or the delivery suite to practise. This is a fantastic opportunity to choose where you would like to learn and gain some further know-how. This experience is then invaluable for future applications and interviews. At the end of your elective, you may even decide that it is not the career path for you – which is fine – it is ideal to know this at this earlier stage of your career.

In summary, think carefully about what department you would like to work in. This will make it easier to plan and structure your placement so that you can focus on that area. If you are undecided, that is fine; you may wish to undertake rotations through several departments. This will assist you with your future career decision-making – even if it helps you to decide where you don't want to work!

What you shouldn't do

I hasten to counsel that you should never be expected to perform procedures for which you are not trained to do. In some countries, you are subject to local student registration, and you should note any requirements contained therein (including not to work unsupervised). If anything were to go wrong, and complications, infections or issues arose, either at the time or at a later stage, a student could be in a difficult situation. As a student, if you wish to assist with procedures, you should ask the local staff to show you and then supervise you. This can be a great learning exercise and good experience. Please understand that mistakes do happen. Patients may be unsatisfied with the outcome and raise issues (whether justified or not).

Therefore, it is important to have a student medical indemnity policy (free for medical students). Student medical indemnity is meant to cover you in the event of an unfortunate situation; however, it may not cover you for performing procedures unsupervised. Therefore, please read and understand the policy document.

If an issue were to occur, do not hesitate to contact your

indemnifier, explain what happened and get their advice. They are experienced in dealing with these issues and negotiating a resolution. For example, a simple letter of apology could be all that is needed to appease an unhappy patient (and their family).

CHAPTER 3

POPULAR DESTINATIONS FOR ELECTIVES

#letsgosomewhere

With so many destinations to choose from, a few of the most popular countries (from my experience with medical students) are discussed below. The focus being on how receptive the hospitals generally are towards welcoming medical students, plus some of the highlights of visiting each country.

Nepal

Nepal is very popular to visit with its unique culture, diversity and dramatic scenery. Explore and go shopping in the colourful streets of Thamel in Kathmandu, breathe in the natural beauty of Pokhara, and go on safari in the Chitwan National Park. Not forgetting the many Buddhist and Hindu temples, and the opportunity to spend a night in a monastery with Buddhist monks. Trekking in Nepal is very popular and there are many treks of varying duration and difficulty to choose from. The food is healthy with plenty of vegetable curries (tarkari), lentil soup (dhal), rice (bhat), spinach (saag), potatoes, and tomato pickle (achar), as well as a delicious array of spices and curries.

Nepal provides a lot of flexibility with placements in departments of your choice across a variety of hospitals. It is also possible to travel to remote clinics and help in remote health camps where there is a real shortage of medical professionals and poor infrastructure makes it difficult for locals to travel to main hospitals. Students can also visit local schools and disabled children's homes to undertake mini-health checks as well as teach health, hygiene and first aid classes or even help them with their English pronunciation and reading.

The doctors in Nepal are very keen to share their knowledge and are happy to teach you new skills. Resources are limited and conditions are difficult; however, the locals maintain a positive attitude. Your new friends at the hospital will often invite you for a trek, and their frequent festivals offer an abundance of music, dance, food and colourful costumes. Get involved in everything and enjoy the unique experience.

Nepal is a relatively cheap place to visit and much of its population live in poverty. There is usually ample capacity for students at many of the hospitals; therefore, it is possible to book a placement in Nepal at short notice.

Fiji

The Fijians are incredibly warm and welcoming. They may seem shy, but they are usually always wearing a big smile. The locals can be a little laid-back (often living on what is called 'Fiji time' or 'island time'), and they value interpersonal relationships more than punctuality. Therefore, it is important to remain patient and build good relationships with the staff.

Many Australians have fond memories of Fijian holidays in the luxury of five-star resorts; however, the reality of living and working in Fiji is a long way from this scene. In any case, students love the opportunity to participate in many water sports, such as snorkelling, visit the beaches and admire the beautiful sunsets.

Most of the guesthouses have self-catering facilities and this provides an ideal opportunity to explore the local market places to buy fresh tropical fruit and vegetables. Visit the supermarkets for your groceries and bottled water.

Staff in the hospitals are very friendly and invite students to get involved in their work as much as possible. The larger hospitals in Suva, Lautoka and Labasa offer all of the main departments. However, the hospitals in Sigatoka, Savusavu and Nadi are smaller and refer serious cases to the larger hospitals. Community medicine is popular at the smaller hospitals and provides the opportunity to visit local villages, homes and schools to provide primary health care to the community. Many students enjoy this experience.

The elective placements are quite restricted, such that you must choose only one department to work in (i.e. medical, surgery, paediatrics, O&G, community medicine, dentistry or physiotherapy). Split placements are not permitted (i.e. your elective can only be in one location), and you are not usually able to choose your preferred location.

Fiji is a very popular choice for medical students (particularly those from colder environments); however, there are simply not enough places (or supervisors) to handle the demand. Students therefore need to book more than 12 months ahead and be flexible on the choice of departments.

Tonga

Tonga is an archipelago in the South Pacific Ocean and is the perfect alternative to Fiji. It has been less popular for students, so it is easier to secure a placement. As a tropical island, Tonga is warm and laidback. The people speak English, and the staff are welcoming.

There is also more flexibility in the Tongan hospitals and so students can choose to rotate through various departments, including surgery, ED, O&G, paediatrics, mental health and general medicine. The main hospital in the capital of Nuku'alofa has 200 beds and around 52 doctors. There are also smaller hospitals on the outer islands that welcome students. They regularly see chronic diseases such as diabetes and heart disease.

There are also community outreach programs (with specific focus on diabetes, dental, medical and health promotion), and these programs are a great opportunity to visit remote villages, homes and health centres.

The people are family oriented and devotedly Christian. Therefore, not much happens on Sundays (other than church). However, enjoy the water activities (canoeing, water skiing, swimming) and the odd invitation to someone's cousin's wedding. Life moves at a slower pace in Tonga, so you can learn to appreciate this way of life and their culture. Shop for fresh fruit and vegetables at the markets and buy your grocery items and bottled water at the corner kiosks that are sprinkled around the town.

Cambodia

Cambodia is a wonderful place to visit that has a beautiful countryside, welcoming people and delicious (and cheap) food. There are plenty of mild curries made with fish, chicken, and vegetables, as well as lots of fresh tropical fruits, mango smoothies and good coffee.

Visiting the Angkor Temples near Siem Reap is an absolute must, and you should aim to spend a full weekend exploring the temples spread across the Angkor Park. Take a boat ride down the Mekong River to the capital of Phnom Penh, and check out the Royal Palace and the colonial architecture. Battambang is the second-largest city and offers unique sightseeing, such as the bat caves, pagodas, numerous temples, and the bamboo train. The local circus (Phare) is not to be missed and is lively entertainment featuring dance, acrobatics, storytelling, and juggling.

Cambodia offers a variety of hospitals across the country. The larger provincial hospitals are government run and provide a wide range of services and departments. However, they are busy, so patient waiting times are long and there are limited resources. Most doctors (not all) speak English, and the patients may be shy – but they are incredibly grateful for anything that you can do for them. Typically, in many Asian hospitals, the family will provide the care for the patients and bring their meals.

The average population is young and many are still affected by the brutal Khmer Rouge regime, which manifests itself in mental health issues in the next generation. The people are working hard to improve access to education to build a better life for themselves and their families.

Typical conditions include trauma (road accidents, falls and landmine injuries), infections (often due to poor hygiene), diabetes, hypertension and malnourishment. Dental, surgical and obstetrics are always busy. Traditional medicine is still practised in remote areas, and when conditions deteriorate due to ancient practices, it can be heartbreaking to see that the only alternative is amputation or death.

It is best to avoid visiting Cambodia during the wet season (June–September) when it can be quite humid and heavy rains may result in some roads becoming flooded.

Sri Lanka

Sri Lanka is a beautiful tropical island with a fascinating history and an interesting variety of temples, forts, national parks, tea planta- tions and stunning surf beaches. Take a safari in the Yala National Park on the weekend and see elephants, leopards and crocodiles. Sri Lankan food is delicious with many curries made from vegetables, lentils, coconut milk, chicken or seafood, and with beautiful blends of herbs and spices. There may be side dishes of pickles and chutneys, best washed down with coffee or a selection of local teas.

There are large teaching hospitals that provide health care on a 24/7 basis. The doctors speak English well; however, they can be demanding and the pace can be frantic. The hospitals are often over-crowded, and many patients do not present until their conditions are quite advanced and thus more complicated to treat.

Medical students often have the opportunity to provide basic health care in community projects such as orphanages, disabled children's homes, or a home for the elderly. These people may not receive proper care or have regular access to a doctor, and therefore it is beneficial for them to have a check-up and learn about health, hygiene and first aid.

Guesthouses and homestays often include meals and this can save a lot of time by not having to prepare and cook your own meals. Travel to work by tuktuk – an entertaining way to travel, although no one can guarantee your safety. Alternative transport options include public buses or walking. Trains are an interesting experience for longer journeys around the country and are incredibly cheap and easy to master. Both trains and buses tend to be quite crowded and the climate is often hot and humid. It is interesting to people-watch – the women dress in brightly coloured saris, and the nurses' uniforms always seem to look impeccable.

Sri Lanka has capacity for many students across its large hospitals; however, it is a destination that you should book well in advance to ensure you have a place. You will also need to arrange your visa a few months ahead and this can be done online.

Tanzania

Tanzania is an amazing destination with its safari parks, Masai warriors, Mount Kilimanjaro, trekking opportunities and coffee plantations. Further afield is the exotic spice island and beautiful beaches of Zanzibar. The people are friendly, and personal relationships are more important than punctuality (much like Fiji!).

As tourists, the local people will assume that you are very

wealthy. Therefore, you should be aware of your personal safety at all times. Do not carry valuables with you, and try to explore the surrounds with other people. I am not suggesting that it is dangerous, it is just important to be prepared and not take unnecessary risks.

Local travel is often via mini-van (dala-dala), which can be crowded, cheap and fun – particularly if you are not tall. You will see many people walking long distances along the roadside at night and this, sadly, brings with it some trauma.

It is a large but crowded country, and there never seems to be enough doctors to cope with the demand for health care. The hospitals offer all the major departments, and it is particularly busy in the emergency and obstetrics departments. There are very limited resources, and patients are expected to pay for diagnostics and buy their own medications.

However, many patients will go without because they simply can't afford it.

Tanzania is also an interesting location for learning more about infectious diseases. There is also a lot of focus on testing, treating and counselling those with HIV. There will be a subtle code on the patient's file in order to avoid embarrassment or stigma for those living with AIDS. HIV exists in many developing countries and therefore it is worthwhile asking the hospital in advance about the precautions and process for managing a needle-stick injury. Hospitals generally have a procedure for the reporting, assessment and management of those with HIV, and many hospitals have PEP in stock. You will probably wish to discuss this with your university staff for their advice and protocol on this issue.

Tanzania is comprised of a wide range of tribes, ethnicities and cultures, and as such the food is usually very diverse. As you would expect in Africa, there is an abundance of game, and the diet contains plenty of meat of many different beasts. Meals are often Indian-style curries, rice, ugali, and chapati. Breakfasts generally consist of Chai (tea), toast, fruit, and mandazi (deep-fried dough). There are also plenty of fruits and nuts to snack on.

Namibia

Namibia is a land of unique beauty. Located on the west coast of sub-Saharan Africa, it is sparsely populated, full of untamed landscapes, tropical forests along rivers, and vast expanses of desert. Its plant and wildlife are tremendously varied, with elephants, cheetahs, mongoose, jackals, meerkats, and over 20 species of antelope all calling this land home.

Namibia's culture is derived from a diverse mix of people. The nation has a proud and fascinating cultural heritage, which is preserved in the form of thriving indigenous communities infused with the customs and traditions of their ancestors.

Despite a shortage of trained medical professionals, government regulations limit access to hospitals for foreign medical volunteers and students. Opportunities are therefore limited to charitable health care clinics that service remote communities. There is often research being undertaken on local conditions and therefore this can be an interesting location for those interested in infectious diseases and research projects.

The medical clinic in Namibia is isolated and about three to four hours from the capital, Windhoek. It serves many small communities of 'the San' people. This group of people are also often referred to as 'the Bushman people', and the clinics are dedicated to their health and welfare. The local people are considered to represent the oldest culture in the world, and they are traditionally hunter-gatherers.

They live in extreme poverty, and so the aim of the medical clinics is to give the next generation the education, health care and help they need to survive and build a brighter, healthier future. It is mainly primary health care that is provided at the clinic, and nearly half of the patients are children. The medical projects conducted in Namibia are therefore of interest to those keen to work in paediatrics, public health, or tropical medicine.

TB and HIV are prevalent in the community. And so the risk of catching TB is managed by ensuring that the clinic is well aired and that the staff have access to face masks. Any patients that are coughing are required to wear masks. Students and volunteers may not be allowed on certain trips if there is a patient with TB travelling in the same ambulance.

A major project conducted by the clinic is the surveys to detect TB. One of the most interesting experiences I have heard about was when a student visited some of those villages for the surveys. On arrival they were met by lots of friendly mothers with their babies and children wanting their photos taken. As well as conducting examinations, a video was shown to them that depicted the signs and symptoms of TB, and the children crowded around to watch it – fascinated by the pictures rather than the message!

Alcoholism, adult onset diabetes, cardiovascular disease, and cataracts and cancer are sharply increasing. Common diseases among the paediatric patients include fungal infections, intestinal worms, diarrhoea, dehydration, malnutrition, and mouth infections. The clinic also assesses and treats emergency patients, and there is, on average, one emergency trip to the hospital each week, which is around one and a half hours drive away. In addition to the clinic, there is regular outreach work at local schools and a resettlement programme. The clinic also distributes donations of clothes, shoes, soap and toothbrushes to adults and children.

Ecuador

Ecuador is one of South America's tiniest countries; however, it is bursting with vibrant and diverse culture, mesmerising landscapes, exotic tropical wildlife and pristine habitats. Part of the massive Amazon jungle lies within Ecuador and is rich in natural resources and home to a wealth of fascinating creatures and indigenous communities.

This country contains a culture that is expressed in an abundance of delicious cuisine, diverse musical forms and colourful festivals. There are remote villages that are extremely poor and without adequate medical assistance and, in many cases, they still use ancient jungle produce to attempt to cure themselves.

Ecuador is a convenient gateway to the Galapagos Islands. Guayaquil is vibrant and boasts a growing arts scene with theatre, film, lively bars and several large universities. The city's riverfront scene is the Malecon that runs along the Rio Guayas. South America is an attractive destination to visit for longer-term electives because it needs plenty of time to soak up the atmosphere and explore the huge continent.

Intermediate-level Spanish skills are required for South American projects (excluding Brazil where Portuguese-speaking skills are required). Students are often keen to learn and practise their Spanish while living and working abroad, and this is a fantastic opportunity to do so. You should not underestimate the importance of learning the language in order to get the most out of your elective. If you feel that time (and energy commitments) spent learning about medicine is more than adequate while you are on your elective, we would not recommend you taking on this additional language-learning workload unless you were really committed to do so.

Lunch is often provided at the hospital while you are at work. For dinner, local specialities, such as lemon-marinated shrimp, ceviche made with fish or seafood, and marinated beefsteak, can be found in cafes and restaurants. Vegetarians are welcome, as there is an extensive range of dishes on offer for non-meat eaters.

You should remain open-minded and flexible with the hospital conditions in Ecuador. You may find it interesting and challenging to resolve issues without the same technology used at home. This will provide you with a comprehensive learning experience while still allowing you plenty of time to see the sights and experience the hustle and bustle of the festivals of the country. Staff are more than happy to help answer questions and make you feel at home in this friendly, vibrant community.

Opportunities available in the various countries

Country	Department						
	General medical	ED	O&G	Surgical	Community Health	Paeds	Rotation
Nepal	✓	✓	✓	✓	✓	✓	✓
Fiji	✓	✓	✓	✓			✓
Tonga	✓	✓	✓	✓	✓		✓
Cambodia	✓	✓	✓	✓	✓	✓	
Sri Lanka	✓	✓	✓	✓	✓	✓	✓
Tanzania	✓	✓	✓	✓		✓	✓
Namibia	✓				✓	✓	
Ecuador	✓			✓		✓	✓

The above matrix provides a general idea of which countries offer more opportunities in the departments that may be of interest to you. If you are interested in a particular country that has not been mentioned, please get in touch with us at DocTours. New destinations with worthwhile placements are added from time to time due to popular requests from students.

SECTION TWO

||||||||||||||||||||||||||||||||||||||||||||||||||||||||||||||||||||||||||||||||||||||||||||||

Preparing and Doing
Your Elective

Once you have decided where to go (or you have narrowed it down to a couple of destinations on your short list), it is time to prepare your application, gather the required documentation needed, and start investigating just what you will be doing on your 'working' adventure. You might be wondering about safety tips, visa requirements and the costs involved in visiting your country of choice.

In this chapter, I have therefore included a pre-departure checklist, suggestions on what to pack, and tips on how to choose suitable accommodation.

I have also collated some recommendations on how to source and present donations of medical supplies to the foreign hospital, as well as elaborated on what you can expect when doing your elective in a developing country, which includes what to do when things go wrong, and what 'fun' you can get up to 'after hours'.

There's a lot to cover, but take it one step at a time and, before you know it, you'll have your elective journey all organised.

CHAPTER 4

PREPARATION

#preparationpreventspoorperformance

Preparing and budgeting for your medical elective overseas is not the sexiest part of the journey, but it is certainly an important aspect of the process.

The application process (and all of the documentation required) takes some time to arrange, and most of these documents will be required whether you are travelling overseas or domestically.

The health and safety tips and suggestions for managing risk are relevant for all travellers, as is the section on budgeting and how to finance your journey.

So, let's get 'prepared'!

Finalising your decision and the application process

As you narrow down your options and preferences for your medical elective, ensure that you apply for a couple of places so that you don't miss out on at least one opportunity. If you book through an arranger, they will usually be able to find something (or anything) at short notice.

Whether you are using an arranger or approaching a hospital directly (or doing both), some of the documents that you will typically need for your application include:

- [ ] A brief CV/resume showing your contact details, your university and course details and dates, any background work experience, volunteer experience, interests and relevant skills (other languages spoken, first aid training, etc.).
- [ ] A letter of 'good standing'. Ask your university course coordinator about how to organise this. It is basically a letter from your university confirming that you are a student in your nominated course, the stages of the course that you have completed, and also confirming that you are required to undertake a clinical placement (and any criteria for the placement). It may take a few weeks to arrange this letter, so I recommend requesting it well in advance.
- [ ] Passport and a passport-sized photo.
- [ ] An application form. This is to obtain personal contact details, next of kin, and details of any allergies or relevant medical conditions.
- [ ] Other forms that may be required. You may be asked to provide a personal reference, a police/criminal background report, or a 'working with children' clearance (or a similar document).
- [ ] Forms that you may also be asked to sign either in advance or when you arrive at your placement include a Code of Conduct and Child Protection Policy.

It may take a month (or longer) to arrange some of the above documents and so it is a good idea to start collating them prior to when you want to submit your applications. There is a lot of paperwork involved (that's life)!

Pre-departure Risk Management Country Risk

I always refer to the Australian Government's Department of Foreign Affairs and Trade (DFAT) safety ratings published on their website: https: smartraveller.gov.au. Their rating system uses four levels of travel advice:

Level 1	Exercise **normal** safety precautions (countries include: Cambodia, Fiji, Tonga, Namibia, Sri Lanka, New Zealand).
Level 2	Exercise a **high degree** of caution (countries include: Nepal, Timor Leste, Ecuador, Tanzania).
Level 3	**Reconsider** your need to travel (countries include: Pakistan, PuertoRico, North Korea).
Level 4	**Do not travel** (countries include: Iraq, Afghanistan, South Sudan).

It is okay to travel to countries that are rated Level 1 or Level 2. You will find that you can easily get travel insurance and medical indemnity cover for your visit to countries in these levels. You will also find that your university is comfortable with you doing your elective in destinations rated Level 1 or 2.

The rating levels change from time to time based on political or civil unrest, or natural disasters such as floods or earthquakes. A natural disaster may affect a small part of the country and therefore you should check carefully on which areas you may be visiting, as well as the ratings of those areas, and then make an informed decision on whether to visit or change your plans or dates.

You can register your travel plans and contact details on the Australian Government's DFAT website: https://orao.dfat.gov.au/pages/secured/default.aspx so that you can be contacted in an emergency (such as natural disaster, civil unrest or family issue), and you can receive free health and safety information. Therefore, please register details of your trip on this site, or the equivalent at your national embassy. You can also subscribe to their updates so that you are aware of emerging risks and plan accordingly.

Countries such as New Zealand, Canada, the USA, and the UK have similar government websites that offer advice and safety information for those travelling overseas – be sure to check out any information your home country offers.

NZ: safetravel.govt.nz
Canada: travel.gc.ca/travelling
USA: wwwnc.cdc.gov/travel/page/survival-guide
UK: www.gov.uk/guidance/foreign-travel-checklist

Insurance

Obtain travel insurance (with unlimited medical evacuation cover) and leave a copy with someone you trust at home. Ensure you have access to the insurance company's 24/7 contact number. Contact your medical professional indemnity provider (or student provider) to advise them of your plans for your elective or international volunteer program. Many will extend free coverage under certain conditions.

Visa

Check on the correct visas required for your elective program and whether you can apply on arrival, or if you need to arrange it before you leave. Ensure that your passport expires at least six months after you return home and that you have some spare blank pages in your passport.

It is very important to have the correct visa (including a transit visa where required), and that you have everything necessary for your visa application. This will include correctly completing the visa application, supplying a recent passport-sized photo, and paying the required fee – usually in USD in cash. Officials will also need to see your passport and your return airline ticket and, occasionally, evidence that you have sufficient funds to support yourself during your stay.

There are penalties for overstaying your visa and for having the incorrect visa. A few years ago, an associate arrived in Tanzania and obtained a tourist visa on arrival. He then attended various meetings with the accommodation providers, and at the hospitals and with the various suppliers that we work with. There have been many changes to the visa and work permit requirements for volunteers in Tanzania over the years, and therefore he raised some questions in one of the more remote locations as to the changes. The well-meaning staff member had a good relationship with immigration and so they visited the local immigration team to discuss the current visa requirements.

During the meeting, the staff member asked about the associate's role and which visa he had obtained. An argument ensued because they were adamant that he was not a 'tourist' and that he was working and should have applied for the (more expensive) Work Permit. He started to get nervous about the potential repercussions of this inadvertent error, and he had visions of receiving a large fine and being thrown into a Tanzanian jail. Being a young male travelling alone, this was not a pleasant thought. The staff member asked if he had his passport with him. The associate lied and said 'no', as he did not want to lose possession of his passport. He then hastily finished the meeting and left the country as soon as he possibly could.

I share this with you to ensure that you do some thorough research into the visa requirements of your chosen country. Note also that visa and work permit requirements can change frequently, and so it's best to check again a few weeks prior to travelling. You do not want to find yourself with the wrong visa when you finally get over there!

Pre-departure health management

It's so important to have your health checked and all necessary health insurance organised before you leave. Focus on the following:

Medical Appointment – See your doctor (or a travel doctor) for advice and to update your travel vaccinations around two to three months prior to travelling overseas. Also ensure that you have a sufficient supply of any prescription medications for your personal use and anti-malarial prophylaxis if required. Useful websites include:

- Australia: smartraveller.gov.au
- NZ: safetravel.govt.nz/staying-healthy-while-travelling
- Canada: travel.gc.ca/travelling/health-safety/vaccines
- USA: wwwnc.cdc.gov/travel
- UK: www.traveldoctor.co.uk

Vaccinations against polio, tetanus, diphtheria, pertussis, measles, mumps, rubella and varicella are normally provided as part of Australia's childhood vaccination program; however, a booster may be required. And if you live in New Zealand, Canada, the USA, or the UK, make sure you check to see what you have been vaccinated for in the past, and if a booster is also required.

If you wear glasses, take a spare pair and/or a copy of the prescription so that they can be replaced more easily if lost or broken.

Travel Insurance – Comprehensive coverage is required with unlimited medical evacuation coverage to protect you in the event of illness or injury. Also note whether you are covered for any pre-existing medical conditions or additional adventure activities (such as paragliding or riding a motorcycle). If you are planning something adventurous, World Nomads (www.worldnomads.com/travel-insurance) provides travel insurance for many of these activities.

Health Risks – Also note on www.smartraveller.gov.au any specific health issues for the countries and regions that you are visiting. The most common health risks in developing countries include high levels of air pollution, altitude sickness, mosquito-borne illnesses (including malaria, dengue fever and Japanese encephalitis), and infectious diseases (including TB and HIV/AIDS).

Infectious diseases – including water-borne, food-borne, parasitic, and others (typhoid, cholera, hepatitis, swine flu, leptospirosis and rabies) – may also be prevalent with serious outbreaks occurring from time to time.

Pack your own masks, gloves and antiseptic hand gel for personal use, as well as your own small first aid kit.

Health tips while overseas

Take precautions to manage these health risks, including wearing masks, insect repellent, long clothing, and take vaccinations/prophylaxis. Also ensure that your accommodation is mosquito proof or you may need to bring a mosquito net.

Maintain good personal hygiene (take and use antiseptic hand gel), and boil all drinking water, or drink bottled water. I do not even brush my teeth using the tap water in some countries. Also avoid ice cubes, and raw or undercooked food.

When choosing restaurants, busier venues with lots of local customers are often a good bet; they will have a higher turnover of food and therefore it is more likely to be fresh and safe. Choose foods and dishes that are freshly cooked using local produce that is in season. (I never order fish in the middle of a desert, as you don't know if it has been kept chilled since it left the water.)

Many other smart travellers choose to eat only vegetarian food in many developing countries to avoid the risk that the meat is not fresh or kept chilled.

Be wary of buffet tables, as the food may have been sitting around for a while at sub-optimal temperatures and could have been visited by flies (or human hands). It is also preferable to peel your own fruits so that you know that it is clean and fresh.

Safety tips while overseas

Your personal safety is paramount; so educate yourself on any and all precautions you can take to ensure a safe and happy trip. Some important aspects to highlight include:

Avoiding Theft – Pickpockets and bag snatchers are relatively common in many developing countries. It is usually fairly obvious that you are a visitor, and therefore you will be perceived to be wealthy, thus making you a target. Do your best to blend in with the locals. Do not take or wear expensive jewellery, and don't place all your valuables in the one bag. Wear the money belt, keep your money out of sight, and lock your valuables in your accommodation (if there is no safe deposit box, then lock items in your luggage where they are out of sight).

Your accommodation hosts can provide useful tips and advice on how to get your bearings and learn to navigate your new neighbourhood safely and with confidence. Try to avoid travelling alone at night, and let your hosts know where you are going and approximately what time you will be home. Keep the numbers of a few reliable taxi drivers stored in your phone.

ATMs and Credit Cards – Fraud and skimming of card details are fairly common; therefore, try to keep your card within sight at all times to ensure that it is not copied. Be wary of using ATMs on the street, alone or at night. It's best to go into a bank to use their ATM.

Avoid Civil Unrest – Be aware of any political demonstrations, elections and protests, and avoid them, as they may turn violent.

Culture and Language – Be mindful of local customs and cultural issues. In particularly, dress conservatively and appropriately for the environment. Understanding key words and phrases of the local language will assist in communicating and learning about imminent dangers.

Be Sensible – Obey the local laws. Do not get involved with drugs, and do not drink excessive quantities of alcohol. Be wary of the hygiene in local tattoo and body piercing parlours.

What it will cost

Budgeting is not always fun. Here is a list of the main items that you will need to buy either before or while travelling overseas. Use the table to fill in your estimates while you are doing your research and planning. Always keep a buffer for the unexpected expenses while travelling.

Item	Where to look	Budget range: $
Flights from home to your destination	Websites such as STA Travel, Expedia, Webjet, and your preferred (or discount) airlines. Flights are generally cheaper if you book well in advance.	
Accommodation	University or hospital on-campus accommodation, homestay, guesthouse, friends, family, BnB or hostel.	
Airport transfers and daily travel to/from hospital/clinic	Public transport options. Ask your accommodation provider for suggestions on how to get around cheaply as a local.	

Meals, bottled water, laundry	Aim to eat like a local. Ask them about the best places to eat that are safe. Buy your bottled water from a supermarket. Some local laundromats may wash, dry and fold your clothes for USD1/kg. Otherwise, use the sink in the bathroom.	
Visa and registration fees	The university or hospital where you are doing your placement may provide some guidance on the appropriate visa, and any registration fees that are applicable. Some visas can be applied for on arrival at the foreign airport, and this is usually the cheapest way to obtain a visa. However, it is essential to check in advance and also reconfirm this information prior to your departure. Contact the nearest embassy or consulate of the country you intend to visit for the latest advice on visa requirements, the cost and the documents required. There are also visa agencies that can process your visa application for you (e.g. CIBT), and they charge an additional fee for their service.	
Passport	Check that your passport expiry date is at least six months after you return home. Obtaining a new passport can take a few months so don't leave it to the last minute! Also carry at least four passport-sized photos with you, as they are often required for your visa and hospital ID card.	
Elective fees	Hospitals and universities may charge an application fee and a weekly fee to cover their costs.	

Professional indemnity insurance or Medical Defence.	MIPS, MDA, MIGA. These organisations provide free indemnity cover for your elective. There are usually exclusions (e.g. they often exclude USA), so check and apply online well in advance.	
Travel insurance	Some indemnity providers (e.g. MIPS) also provide free travel insurance coverage for student members on their elective. Coverage provides for loss of baggage, travel documents and credit cards, as well as medical expenses. Your university may also arrange coverage for all of their students on an international elective, so check and ensure that you have details of the policy (e.g. phone number and policy number), in case you need it.	
Medical kit	Take your personal first aid kit with a supply of bandages, analgesics, Gastro-Stop, motion sickness meds, as well as your usual medications.	
Vaccinations and malaria prophylaxis	Consult a travel doctor and/or Travelvax. com.au for advice on what is required for your specific destination.	
Spending money and contingencies	Sightseeing, souvenirs, gifts and eating out. Try to keep a secret stash of US$100+ and a credit card for the unforeseen flight delay or departure tax that you were not expecting.	

How to finance the journey

An overseas elective should be one of the most memorable highlights of your medical training. However, figuring out how to pay for the journey (in addition to all of your existing expenses) can cause a bit of anxiety. Therefore, here are a few suggestions on where to source some additional funding:

- Australian Government Loan: OS-HELP is a loan available to eligible students who want to undertake some of their study overseas. The loan can be used for flights, accommodation and other travel or study expenses. To be eligible you must be an Australian citizen with a tax file number and be undertaking full-time study overseas that will be counted towards the requirement of your course (includes clinical placements). In 2019, the maximum amount you could borrow was $6791 (and $8149 if you study in Asia). You repay your loan through the taxation system once your income is above a certain threshold ($51,957 p.a. for the 2018–19 income year), and your repayments are calculated as a percentage of your income (starts at 2% and increases to 8% as your salary increases). There is no interest charged on HELP loans; however, the debt is subject to indexation (measured by the Consumer Price Index).
- Scholarships: It is worthwhile applying for relevant scholarships, particularly if you have a strong academic record or come from a disadvantaged background. Your university may have a database of opportunities available to you, and also have a look at the websites of the various Medical Defence Organisations (MDOs) to see what is available. For example, MIGA has an Elective Grants Program to provide financial assistance to students undertaking their elective in a developing community. There are ten grants annually of $3000, each of which $1500 can assist with travel, accommodation and vaccination costs, and the balance of $1500 can assist with the purchase of medical aid for the community visited.
- Organisations such as MSAP (Medical Student Aid Program) give monetary grants (up to $2000) to Fifth Year medical

students on elective in developing countries to be spent on health resources. AirborneAid recycles and donates unwanted equipment and medical supplies. The purpose is to provide tangible items to improve health outcomes, and it also helps students to make a lasting difference during their elective placement.

- Crowdfunding: The introduction of the online crowdfunding platforms (such as MyCause, Chuffed, and GoFundMe) enables you to approach a wider audience of family, friends and interested parties. They can help share the cost of your once-in-a-lifetime experience, particularly if you highlight the positive social impact of visiting and helping in a developing country.
- Borrow from a financier. Banks such as the Bank of Queensland provide a short-term overdraft facility to help bridge the gap between your savings and other funding sources, such as the government loan or a scholarship.
- Your 'parent's bank'.

CHAPTER 5

PLANNING YOUR JOURNEY

#travelplans

You have made the important decision about where to go, your placement has been confirmed, and your departure date is rapidly approaching. You probably have exams and assessments to focus on; however, you have the excitement of your overseas adventure to look forward to.

To save you time, I have provided you with a pre-departure checklist, suggestions on what to pack, what to wear, and how to manage donations of any medical supplies that you may wish to take. I have also included my top tips on how to choose suitable accommodation.

Essential pre-departure information

Your pre-departure checklist should include the following:

✓ **Flights** – Book online directly with the airline, a travel website or an online travel agency.

✓ **Arrival Transfer** – I recommend that you organise an airport arrival transfer in advance. You may arrive in a foreign city late at night and be tired and jet-lagged. Therefore, it is much safer (particularly if you have not been to that country recently) to have someone reputable meet you and transfer you to your pre-booked accommodation.

✓ *Embassy Registration* – Your home country embassy may contact you in case of an emergency and can provide free health and safety information. Therefore, please register details of your trip on www.smartraveller.gov.au (if your home country is Australia), or the equivalent at your national embassy.

✓ *Vaccinations* – See your doctor (or a travel doctor) around two to three months prior to travelling overseas for advice on travel vaccinations.

✓ *Travel Insurance* – Obtain travel insurance (with unlimited medical evacuation cover) and leave a copy with someone you trust.

✓ *MDO* – Contact your medical indemnity provider to advise them of your plans for your elective.

✓ *Visa* – Check on the correct visas required for your elective and whether you can apply on arrival.

✓ *Pack Your Bag* – Try to travel light and note the limits on carrying liquids in your hand luggage. Do some reading on the country that you are visiting and learn some of the local language. Take some US dollars – it's recommended to take small denominations, and some countries may only accept new notes that are in good condition. Arrange a SIM card upon your arrival or talk to your network provider before you leave about their international travel plans.

Items to pack, take and wear

One of the most frequently asked questions is: 'What do I wear?' Staff in developing countries are often surprised at this question. Perhaps it is not important to them, and their response may be 'just come as you are'. For us, we don't want to offend, and we like to blend in, be part of the team, and often we feel accepted if we are wearing the right gear.

Many developing countries still expect doctors and medical students (and often nurses) to wear a white coat. In Cambodia and Nepal, all the doctors and medical students wear a white coat, as it's an easy way for patients to identify the various people in the hospital and their roles.

One volunteer nurse was working in the emergency department in Nepal. On her first day they received a trauma patient. She wrote: 'First day down and it was full on. Within ten minutes of arriving, the white coat had to go, as we had a trauma and got covered in blood!'

The Packing List – I have collated a list of recommendations and suggestions, but of course it is up to you. Firstly, check the season and the weather forecast at your destination. Remember not to pack fluid/paste in a container larger than 100ml in your hand luggage. All liquids must be in a clear plastic bag for security clearance at the airport.

Here's a list of other items to include:

The Packing List

For clinical placements: scrubs or white coat, or conservative lightweight cotton skirts, dresses, trousers and shirts. Comfortable, closed-toe shoes. Scrubs are recommended for village visits and outreach work, as there is a need to be flexible, and you will definitely get dirty!

	Shorts, T-shirts, sandals/flip flops, modest swimsuit, PJ's, light clothes for relaxing at night, windbreaker or lightweight raincoat. Layers of clothes are handy for colder climates, or if it gets colder at night.
	Sarong – also useful to wear while working in the remote villages.
	Copies of all travel documents and contact information. Leave a copy at home with someone trustworthy.
	Alarm clock
	Earplugs
	Money belt or passport pouch
	Prescription medication
	Contact lens solutions
	Water bottle
	Towels
	Toothbrush/toothpaste
	Shampoo, conditioner
	Tissues, toilet paper and sanitary items. Many developing countries do not provide toilet paper, so it is always handy to have your own supply. Importantly, do not flush paper down the toilet – most Asian plumbing cannot cope with these items being flushed, so please place paper and used sanitary items into the bin next to the toilet.
	Phone, camera and charger
	Small umbrella
	Sunglasses and hat
	Bug spray and bug bite cream. It is also a good idea to use fragrance-free toiletries.
	Sunscreen

	Torch/flashlight
	E-books/magazines/iPod/iPad or DVDs (optional)
	Charger or two for your devices, plus an international/universal electrical plug
	Pen and paper for taking notes at work
	For weekend travel and sporting activities, take a smaller backpack and travel towel, sturdy foot wear for walks, as well as long pants and light, long-sleeved shirts for protection.
	Leave all valuable items at home – there is no need for designer goods or expensive jewellery.
	Take a padlock or combination lock to keep items locked safely in your suitcase.
	Take a copy of your CV, passport, airline ticket, credit cards and any medical registration documents with you, plus a stethoscope.
	Take some disposable gloves, face masks and hand sanitiser for your use.

Documents and items to take in your hand luggage

Take recent copies of your resume, airline tickets, travel insurance, passport, and some spare passport-sized photos with you in your hand luggage. Carry some USD cash with you – it is internationally recognised and readily accepted. Wear a money belt even when you are on the plane, for your cash, debit/credit cards and travel documents. I always pack an empty water bottle in my hand luggage and then refill it regularly on the plane. And I suggest you also pack a book on the country you are visiting, or some language books to study, as these will keep you entertained while you travel.

Taking donations of medical supplies

It is recommended that you ask your chosen hospital in advance as to what equipment and supplies they are lacking and bring these items if you can. Many students and volunteers report shortages of sterile gloves, analgesic medications, and antibiotics.

Most people travel to Nepal with their own gloves, hand-rubs, stethoscope, disposable aprons (useful when attending wound dressings), disposable masks, scissors, tapes (micropores), crepe bandages, and Band-Aids. You should bring your own BP set (sphygmomanometer) and stethoscope as in many developing countries the wards will not have extra sets.

When an orthopaedic ward's BP stethoscope didn't work in a remote hospital in Nepal, they had to borrow from general surgery! There was only one ECG machine in ICU, and they lacked the medical 'luxuries' found in Australia and other developed countries.

Donations of clothing and blankets are often delivered to local schools in many developing countries, and the children are delighted to receive new, warm clothes. Undamaged shoes are usually a good donation as well.

Many students suggest taking cannulas, antibiotics and thermometers. They generally need gloves, hand sanitisers, medications, antibiotics and pain relief. It is often possible to buy most of these items abroad – it can actually be quite cheap to do so, and it helps their economy as well.

We suggest that if you are planning to take and donate medical supplies, please follow these guidelines:

- Take them with you on the same flight. Preferably pack them in the bottom of your suitcase. One young nurse travelled to Cambodia with two suitcases – one with her personal items and the other was filled with donations. Unfortunately, the bag full of donations arrived on a different flight, and so she returned to Airport Customs the following day to collect the bag and answer questions about the contents and their value. This is an inconvenience that is best avoided.

- Expiry dates: I do not recommend taking medications that have expired. However, it is generally okay to take donations of bandages and sealed supplies that are near or just past their use-by dates. We have seen many patients in poor countries who can't afford these items and often go without. Therefore, expired bandages are better than none at all. Similarly, I have also seen hospitals in some countries routinely washing and re-using many consumables, and therefore it is better to have new supplies (even if they have passed their 'best before' date).

- Further to the above comments about expiry dates, it is always good to check with hospital staff that work in the specific country before you take expired items overseas. Some countries frown upon the practice (due to a sense of pride?) and will confiscate expired items if they see them (either at the airport or at the hospital/clinic). It then becomes a burden for the country to dispose of the unwanted goods. Some volunteers remove or cover the expiry date or use-by dates on bandages.

Another unfortunate student posted donations to Nepal before she left Australia. She said, 'I made the mistake of posting medical supplies. Next time I won't do this, as they said I had to pay US$500 in tax (the items were valued at around this amount in Australia – i.e. 100% tax).' The posted package had a Customs declaration enclosed that stated the value of the goods.

This is another good example of why we suggest that you take donated items *with you* on the same flight. If you declare them at Customs, the value should always be 'nil' (because they have been donated). It is crazy to pay duty on importing these items, and it is less likely to occur if you are carrying them with you (rather than posting them or having them arrive as unaccompanied luggage). Many charities and humanitarian causes (e.g. the Australian Government, Red Cross, Rotary International, etc.) arrange for container loads of medical equipment and new supplies to be donated to developing countries. I applaud this. However, if there are excess first aid items and expired dressings that you can fit in your suitcase and personally deliver to the hospital while you are there, it is certainly appreciated. It also reduces wastage and results in less landfill at home!

Accommodation options

The internet is fabulous for researching cheap places to stay and comparing photographs of each. A room might look attractive on the website and *seem* to receive rave reviews; however, disappointment could arise because the accommodation or your room is poorly located or noisy. So make sure you read *all* the reviews that are offered. And do several 'searches' on your accommodation of interest across various sites, and ask for recommendations from recent travellers.

The two most popular accommodation styles available for you are either staying in a 'guesthouse' (similar to a private hotel), or as a 'homestay' (staying in someone's home).

'Guesthouse' checklist (and key questions to ask in advance)

With the above issues in mind, and knowing that you are staying in the same room for four to eight weeks, I have developed a checklist of some factors to consider when selecting your guesthouse accommodation. Here's what to look for:

☐ What is the name, address and website of the guesthouse?
☐ Is there a TV? For some people, this is a good way to relax and wind down after a busy or stressful day at the hospital, so make sure you have one to use.

59

☐ Is the room safe for keeping your passport, cash, cards, camera, laptop, etc? If there is no in-room safe, the front desk may have a large safe where you can store your valuables.

☐ Is there air-conditioning and/or a fan? A fan is often more useful for the hot, humid climate in many developing countries.

☐ Is the room cleaned and the linen changed frequently? This is not a major issue; however, it is good to know so that you are aware of when housekeeping may be entering your room. We recommend not leaving any personal or valuable items on display, as it can be tempting, and so it's best to hide them in your suitcase and lock it.

☐ Do the staff speak English? It is important that someone on site speaks your language – particularly in the event of any emergency, and if you need to receive urgent safety instructions. I like to choose a guesthouse that is owned and managed by a family (they may be Westerners, or locals who are very experienced in hosting international guests), as they seem to take care of everything. Families usually take more of an interest in you and are happy to provide advice and information on the local area.

☐ Is there enough cupboard space/storage? When you are living in a particular room for four to eight weeks, you will want to unpack your suitcase, hang up clothes, store all your items, etc.

☐ Are there any laundry facilities? Laundry can get expensive over a four-week period, so it is good to know the options available. You may be happy to wash your underwear and scrubs in the basin and hang them to dry (drying does not take very long in most developing countries, even in winter). There might be a nearby laundromat where you can drop off a bag of dirty clothes in the morning and pick it up that evening at a cost of around US$1–2/kg. Occasionally, there could be a laundry service in-house that is complimentary, so you could take your own laundry detergent. I avoid ironing whenever I am travelling; however, some people like to iron clothes/scrubs, and so they ask in advance if they have access to ironing facilities. You may use a combination of these methods – whatever you decide, it is good to know what is available in advance.

☐ What is the bathroom (basin/shower/loo) like? Knowing if you have your own ensuite bathroom or whether you will be sharing one can affect the price of your accommodation. If sharing, you obviously need to take and wear appropriate nightwear and thongs for traipsing to/from the bathroom.

☐ Is there hot water? Many places advertise and advise that they have 'hot water'; however, this may not always be the case. If there is a shortage of hot water for any reason, I find it easier to tolerate a cool shower during the heat of the afternoon rather than first thing in the morning.

☐ What is the quality of linen and toiletries like? Check if you need to pack your own towels and toiletries. Some people travel everywhere with their own pillow, towel and preferred shampoo. Others, like myself, are happy to use whatever the guesthouse provides.

☐ Is there any Wi-Fi/free internet? Connectivity is the most sought-after item when travelling, and it can get expensive if you get it wrong. Some guesthouses advertise that they have guest Wi-Fi; however, it can actually be incredibly slow and unreliable. I recommend buying a SIM card on arrival, to use for data and talk time. Always ensure that the SIM is correctly registered and working before you leave the store. Alternatively, your phone provider may conveniently offer travel plans for some countries, and so it's worthwhile checking prior to travel, as it could be more expensive than buying a local SIM.

☐ Is there a back-up generator? The electricity (and water)

supply can also be unreliable in developing countries, and so it is good to ask how frequently outages may occur and what contingencies are in place. I also recommend taking a battery-operated torch.

☐ What meals and drinks are available? One of the exciting things about travel is trying the local cuisine. Some guesthouses may provide a kitchenette, so you can prepare your own meals if you prefer to do this. However, keep in mind that developing countries do not have the extensive range of pre-prepared foods at the supermarket that you enjoy at home. You can, however, experience the novelty of visiting a local market place in the town centre that sells fruit, vegetables, fish, fresh meat and spices, and then cook everything from scratch! In some countries, the variety and quality of local cafes and restaurants provides an opportunity to eat out quite cheaply. For example, the Noodle Man in Battambang (Cambodia) will serve a steaming hot bowl of noodles and vegetables in a broth with your choice of meat for around USD60 cents.

☐ What are the guesthouse facility opening hours? Some nights you may wish to relax and eat your dinner in your room. Therefore, it is good to know if this is possible, as well as knowing the opening hours of your guesthouse dining facility and the approximate costs of eating there.

☐ Is breakfast included? Most guesthouses will provide breakfast, and it is wise to check what is available and what time it is available. You may need to depart early for work, so it's a good idea to know that you can eat something before you leave for your day.

☐ Is there a fridge in your room? Long-term visitors like to be able to store their drinks and fruits in their own fridge so that they can access a snack at any time. If there is no fridge in your room, you may wish to ask if there is a shared fridge available for guests.

☐ Are there jug and tea-making facilities? This is a must if you wish to enjoy a hot tea or coffee at any time!

☐ Is your room non-smoking? Many people in Australia, New Zealand, Canada, the USA, and the UK have become quite health-conscious in recent years, and the number of smokers has reduced. However, this is not necessarily the case among people in Asia and Europe. If you are sensitive to cigarette smoke, it is wise to request a non-smoking room.

☐ Is bottled water available? Many facilities will provide one half-litre bottle of water per day; however, you will need at least one to two litres per day for drinking and brushing your teeth. As a reminder, please do not drink tap water in developing countries! Do not even brush your teeth with it! It is good to check the cost of additional water or plan to buy at a local supermarket if it works out cheaper. In the hotter climates, it is important that you do not run out of water. It may be possible to access a large tank of drinking water and then refill your own smaller bottle as needed. This reduces the amount of disposable plastics and is better for the environment.

☐ What is the safety and security like? I recommend that you leave all valuables at home, as there is no need to wear expensive jewellery or designer clothing while travelling on your elective. You may want to take a good camera, a smart phone and a laptop, but keep these in sight at all times. If you are sharing a room with other people (some that you have never met), you should aim to lock your suitcase or access a safe deposit box for your passport, spare cash, credit cards, etc. Some people like to lock their suitcase and attach it to their bed (using a larger padlock or 'handcuffs'). If you are travelling alone, it is good to know about the security arrangements at the guesthouse. For example, it might be a gated community and there could be a security guard or an onsite manager available at all times.

☐ Is there a swimming pool? It is nice to have a refreshing swim after work in the hotter climates. Some guesthouses will have a pool, and others may have access to a pool at a sister property, or they can recommend the local public baths and provide instructions on how to get there.

☐ Is there a communal area? This may include a lounge, TV room, a quiet reading area, pool and bar area. This extra space is ideal for meeting other international travellers and relaxing, so you are not confined to your bedroom.

☐ What is the location? This is a huge consideration. You may want to be close to the hospital where you are working; however, you should investigate whether the location is safe, noisy, or close to public transport. There could be fairly cheap bus services, tuktuks or bicycles that you can access. Developing countries can be notoriously noisy – there always seems to be a rooster crowing before dawn, dogs barking, traffic noise (bikes, trucks, and everything else at all hours), general noise of staff talking, and the noise of equipment being used around the property. If you are a light sleeper, take earplugs and ask for a quiet room. Other factors for location include proximity to a local supermarket, cafes and restaurants, laundry, etc. – ideally so that you can walk to various places.

'Homestay' checklist (and key questions to ask in advance – see above for further details on similar topics)

☐ What is the name, address, and social media site/website of the homestay?
☐ Is there a TV for visitors with English channels?
☐ Is the room safe for keeping valuables?
☐ How many people share a bedroom?
☐ Is there air-conditioning and/or a fan?

☐ How frequently is the room cleaned and the linen changed?
☐ How well do the host family speak English?
☐ Is there enough cupboard space/storage?
☐ Are there any laundry facilities?
☐ What is the bathroom (basin/shower/loo) like? How many people will share the bathroom?
☐ Is there hot water?
☐ What do I need to bring (e.g. towel, linen and toiletries)?
☐ Is there any Wi-Fi/free internet, and is it fast and reliable?
☐ What meals and drinks are available? If you are in a homestay, they often provide all of the meals for you. This is great because it can save you a lot of time in planning, shopping, preparing and cooking the meals.
☐ How flexible are the family if you would like to eat dinner out?
☐ Are you able to use the jug and tea-making facilities at any time?
☐ Is the home and your room non-smoking?
☐ Is bottled water available for drinking and brushing your teeth?
☐ What is the safety and security like?
☐ Is there a communal area?
☐ What is the location?

Perspectives on guesthouse vs. homestay

From my experience, having stayed in the following various countries over the last ten years, I have found that they all have something to offer, and it really depends on the type of experience you wish to have while on your overseas elective.

Guesthouse – In Tonga, the guesthouse accommodation was homely and welcoming; the hosts showed the same Tongan hospitality that I had come to know and enjoy from the locals.

Guesthouse accommodation in Cambodia was excellent – although the internet was a bit slow. Apart from that, it catered for everything amazingly. It was very pleasant having a smaller 'homey' villa for the month, compared to staying in a big hotel.

I especially enjoyed my stay in the 'Volunteer House' in Tanzania, more than expected. My housemates were from many different countries and their ages ranged from 17 to late 50s, and they were volunteering in schools, orphanages, and environmental programs. We had a beautiful view of Mount Kilimanjaro, and there was plenty of time for chatting and getting to know this vast array of people.

The staff were locals, and so I was able to learn from them about the local culture and attitudes, which I greatly appreciated. It gave me a different perspective on life in the country that I wouldn't have been privy to had I just been another tourist. I loved sampling the local food and enjoyed picking fresh mangoes and avocados to accompany my breakfast.

Homestays – A homestay experience can be hugely rewarding. The homestay provides a unique and special insight into the country by combining cultural events, festivals and local knowledge with an elective or volunteering program.

Well-chosen hosts will make you feel a part of their family, welcoming you into their home and providing the support and opportunities to make your trip one that you will never forget. Hosts go that extra mile to ensure the program goes smoothly, accompanying you for your first day at the hospital, as well as to the community outreach programs.

Your host mum's cooking is often incredible. They will usually make delicious home-cooked meals every day, including traditional food. You might even find that they will be keen to teach you how to make some traditional dishes.

In Nepal, most students have reported that their host families were great, and that they served nice food and maintained contact with them via email or social media after they returned home. The hosts often speak English well and engage in some good discussions.

However, one volunteer was based in a more remote homestay and said that his hosts did not speak English and were silent most of the time. He did not feel comfortable and secretly left his room to take a shower after everyone else had gone to bed. The house was located next door to an Indian temple, which was noisy at 4.30 in the mornings.

The homestay hosts in Tanzania were obviously very wealthy, and they often worked late in their export/import business. The home was large and comfortable, and there were several domestic staff. Volunteers had their own room and bathroom; however, only cold showers were available. Situated in close proximity to a church and a mosque made it noisy at night (bells, singing, chanting, etc.). It was about one hour walk to the hospital.

Most students have a fabulous experience with homestay accommodation and appreciate the additional support, new friendships, and the enhanced cultural insights that this type of accommodation offers.

Whichever option you choose, it is worthwhile doing some thorough research so that your experience is a positive one and aligned with your personal preferences.

CHAPTER 6

DOING YOUR ELECTIVE PROGRAM

#adventure

It is your first day at work – time to meet your new colleagues and the patients, as the fun is about to begin. So let's cover what you should do on arrival, how best to communicate with your team, build relationships and trust with your supervisors, work with limited resources, and of course figure out what you should be doing ...

Arrival and orientation

After your placement is confirmed, you will receive more information such as your supervisor's name, working hours and where to go on the first morning. On your first day, there may be paperwork and photo ID to finalise. You will also want a tour of the hospital to get a feel for the location of each department, patients, resources, facilities, administration, meeting rooms, bathroom, tearoom etc. If it is quiet, seek out any handbooks of common conditions and available treatments, as this will always be a useful resource.

Be sure to introduce yourself to the Medical Superintendent (MS) of the hospital, if the opportunity arises. Let him/her know your name, where you are from, your university and the stage you are in your course, as well as how long you are there and if you have any particular areas of interest. Making friends with the assistant (and, in fact, all staff) is a great idea, as they can be a wealth of information and your new best friend.

In an ideal world, your orientation will all happen smoothly and efficiently. In reality, however, it can be a bit of a shemozzle for the first day or so. Paperwork seems to go missing, supervisors get sick or need to be elsewhere, there may be a public holiday, and no one seems to know what is meant to be happening. Don't worry, just smile and be patient.

Be sure to express appreciation for them hosting you during your placement. Tell them how you are looking forward to learning and helping out, as well as communicate any university requirements or paperwork that you need to have signed. Similarly, at the end of your placement, be sure to say thank you and goodbye to all of the staff.

Typically, your working day will be from around 8 am to 4.30 pm from Monday to Friday. If you would like to work extra hours to gain additional knowledge or experience in a particular area, then ask the MS or your supervisor directly, as they can help make it happen. This is particularly relevant for obstetrics, emergency, and surgeries, as one can't plan ahead for these! Similarly, if you want some time off (for a longer weekend excursion or if you are feeling unwell), advise the MS, your supervisor and/or the admin assistant. Otherwise they will worry about where you are and it leaves a bad impression.

What you will see and what you will be doing

Each morning, plan to attend the doctors' handover meeting where there will be discussions about the previous night's admissions, interesting cases, as well as any critical incidents/deaths. Listening to the discussions about the various cases and hearing them challenge certain practices should be a great educational experience, and you could have the opportunity to ask questions as well.

After the meeting, join the doctors on ward rounds, consults, and seeing to outpatients, as this should also provide powerful insights into the health challenges in the community. Most commonly, there will be extreme poverty, limited education and medical options, and so most patients present to the hospital at a very late stage of illness.

The doctors might also head to the hospital canteen or staff tearoom for breakfast/coffee break. If so, be sure to join them and engage in conversation. They are only too willing to discuss interesting cases and give you some tips and advice on getting around.

What to expect at a Nepali ...

Hospital – I once joined a group of medical students on their elective program in Nepal. We slipped off our shoes at the meeting room door at 8.30 am and then the day kicked off with a handover meeting. All of the doctors from the night shift and the heads of departments were present.

Typical conditions that presented overnight included febrile convulsions, pneumonia, UTIs, labour complications, and alcohol poisoning. Occasionally X-ray films were passed around for everyone to review, and there were always constructive discussions about how to handle each case.

The doctors were bright and talented; however, in some cases, they were still young and inexperienced. The chief administrator of the hospital was a retired emergency physician from the US Military. His career spanned six countries, including Antarctica, and he offered great leadership, maturity and fresh ideas for improving communication skills among the staff. Following the morning meeting, students split into groups of three and attached themselves to one of the consultants for ward rounds.

This was followed by a tea break in the hospital canteen. The canteen was similar to an outdoor treehouse, and it was situated on an elevated platform with the most amazing views over the Kathmandu Valley. Over coffee, one of the young doctors explained the complexity involved in cleaning out a deep flesh wound caused by a water buffalo attack to the groin of one of his patients.

Conditions such as hypertension, ischaemic heart disease, chronic obstructive pulmonary disease (COPD), and diabetes are all common, and there is limited access to medication (or many are non-compliant). As a result, many presentations to the hospital are the outcomes of these diseases, including myocardial infarction, stroke and pneumonia. Infectious diseases are also a major challenge, with tuberculosis and typhoid being common causes for admission, as well as septicaemia (mostly from pneumonia). Attempted suicide by organophosphate poisoning is also common.

Clinical acumen is required because the range of investigations and treatment options are limited by availability and cost. However, late presentation and advanced disease means physical signs are often quite pronounced. Patients pay for any treatment, often upfront, and there is no insurance. While the costs are comparatively low by Western standards, they represent a major expenditure for the local people.

Simple tests, including full blood count, electrolytes, renal function, blood cultures and liver function, are available at larger hospitals, as are plain X-rays and ultrasounds, with echocardiography (excluding Doppler) available once a week. CT scans are available at a location 30 minutes away, but they cost US$200.

Medication choices vary depending on availability from suppliers, but most that are relatively cheap and commonly used can be provided. Interestingly, patients usually request and receive almost no analgesia.

Emergency medicine is not currently recognised as a specialised discipline in Nepal, even though they commonly receive trauma, infections, and the complications of chronic disease as well as pregnancy.

Obstetrics departments are busy, and most patients delivering receive antenatal care, helping to keep C-sections to around 15 percent. However, there is a large number of women not receiving antenatal care and delivering at home unsupervised.

Clinical problems faced by the paediatric department include multiple infectious diseases similar to those seen in adults, including tuberculosis, typhoid, hepatitis A and pneumonia. On my visit, some children appeared small and undernourished.

Remote Clinic – Some students who had recently commenced their clinical years arrived in Nepal with little procedural experience. They were therefore mainly keen observers and they learnt far more than they had planned or thought possible. With limited access to specialist facilities, medicine was done as they had read in Talley and O'Connor (the art of diagnosing on clinical knowledge). They praised the local doctors who were incredible teachers and wonderful people.

They were given the opportunity to help out at a rural medical camp. The camp provides women in remote locations access to health care and a chance to see a doctor. There was an early morning start, and they were packed into the back of the van along with medications and some medical equipment. The journey provided time to appreciate the phenomenal landscape.

On arrival, the rooms were organised and the day commemorated with speeches from the village elder. Initially, there seemed to be only a few women waiting; however, they arrived in their hundreds by lunchtime. At the end of the day, they visited one of the villager's homes, enjoying the gracious hospitality of the Nepalese. A thatched mud hut with a low ceiling and a dimly lantern-lit room offered shelter from the summer heat. The students sat barefoot and cross-legged on the cool clay while enjoying a meal with the host and his family. That afternoon topped the students' lists of memories in Nepal.

Emergency Department (ED) – In the larger EDs, patients are often received in more severely critical conditions. There are lots of road traffic accidents, Chronic Obstructive Pulmonary Disease (COPD) with oxygen saturations below 70 percent, patients in altered conscious states, and PV bleeding. Medical students have assisted in resuscitations, doing compressions, assisting with ventilations, and analysing the ECG.

It may be challenging to find your feet initially because the doctors are extremely busy and have less time to explain or translate for you. However, introducing yourself to an intern can be beneficial by having a familiar face and creating a great learning experience.

A smaller ED may have only five beds, one doctor and two to three nurses at a time. However, it can be a more supportive environment to participate in, as the doctors are often eager to teach, explain and answer any questions, as well as translate when taking a patient's history.

Get involved in full patient assessments (to a limited extent due to language barrier), discuss differential diagnosis and potential management options, and take part in handovers to specialties such as paediatrics/orthopaedics. Look at countless chest X-rays, listen to hundreds of chests, assist in the application of casts, administer medication, and help out wherever you can.

Patients walk into the ED and if there is a bed available, they can use it. The system of triage is not well developed. Before a patient is seen by a doctor and any treatment administered, they (or a family member) must pay and then show the receipt to staff.

Patients also need to pay for and collect their meds from the hospital pharmacy to be administered.

Students in the past have spent time at a major trauma centre attached to the plastic surgery and burns ward. Being invited to the operating room to observe and assist during the surgeries has been 'an amazing experience'.

One student said, 'I'm currently three weeks into a four-week placement in Nepal, and I can safely say that I've loved every minute here. I've been exposed to a variety of surgical medicine at two hospitals. In both hospitals, I was welcomed into the out-patient clinic as well as the operating room, and I was made to feel a part of the team despite the language barrier between myself and the patients.'

Obstetrics and Gynaecology (O&G) – Students with a particular interest in women's health have assisted the obstetricians with consults (checking the heartbeat of the foetus, measuring fundus, checking for lymphedema). They have also had the opportunity to observe births, assist in the Operating Theatre (OT) with C-sections and also with incomplete abortions, as well as partic-ipate in antenatal and gynaecological clinics.

Students are often surprised at the lack of privacy between patients and the differences in deliveries between developed countries and Nepal. However, they often feel that they have had incredible exposure in their chosen medical field and report that they would never have had that access back home.

Dermatology – Some students spent time in the dermatology outpatient clinic where patients came for common complaints such as scabies, tinea, abscesses and candidiasis. The dermatolo-gist spent a lot of time explaining the consults and made sure the students were following what was happening. One of the issues was that many medications were available over the counter

(OTC), whereas they would usually require a prescription in a developed country. As a result of this, patients could be buying the wrong medication and potentially worsening their lesions.

A dermatology registrar volunteered in a Plastic and Burns Unit and had a fascinating experience. She was amazed at how they could manage all the lesions with limited resources. As well as assisting the staff, she had the feeling that she was there to learn. She felt really welcomed and comfortable in the hospital. At the completion of her experience, she looked back and realised how much she had learnt and developed, such as working in a team, communicating with people by just looking at their faces, and trying to work with limited resources, which was definitely an overwhelming experience.

What to expect at a Cambodian ...

Hospital – On interviewing several medical students about their experiences while working in hospitals in Cambodia, one medical student told me, 'I was assisting in theatre and practising basic skills such as primary assessment, suturing, and inserting cannulas and catheters.'

Another dental student mentioned that, 'I arrived at the hospital early on Monday morning and was warmly received by the staff in the dental clinic. I observed how everything worked – the patients were called in by the assistant and they took their shoes off at the entrance. They sat in the dental chair and rinsed their mouths before the dentist looked at them. The dental decay and periodontal disease was vast. The severity and prevalence of decay was much higher than I'd seen previously, and it ranged across all ages. One dentist explained that there was no awareness or attempt to explain the importance of oral hygiene. Once the treatment finished, the patient paid their fee with the assistant. The fee was subsided, as it was a government hospital.

From the afternoon on the first day onwards, I was assisting with treatment: extractions, fillings, fractured teeth.'

Clinic – You can expect to see a lot of skin conditions, HPT, diabetes, TB, HIV, malnutrition, coughs and colds, mumps, TB post chemoprophylaxis, upper respiratory infections, diabetic foot ulcers and a variety of other infective wounds that are usually on lower limbs, anaemia, fractures, and complications of other disorders, inclusive of land mine injuries.

Sadly, the Cambodians rarely continue immunisation started at 'baby check' time if born in hospital. There are usually a lot of diabetics to review; however, not many patients use insulin. There are generally a lot of severe secondary infections of injured and burnt limbs, some with probable underlying osteomyelitis. You may even have the opportunity to travel into rural areas to give antibiotic infusions and monitor young patients who probably have leprosy.

The most challenging aspect for many students is the emotional impact of seeing extreme poverty and low living standards. It is also challenging due to the need to rely on clinical skills rather than investigations (due to the cost), or difficulty in gaining an understanding of the patient's complete medical history, as well as the fact that there is no clear referral process (as there is often nowhere to refer them to!). Some students recommend taking a basic medical text, e.g. the *Oxford Handbook*, an otoscope and stethoscope, and jump at the opportunity to visit a hospital and go along on home visits, which are quite confronting due to the poor conditions.

Culture dictates that patients will often attend a traditional healer initially and only go to the clinic when they have more serious problems. An extreme example of this occurred when a patient arrived at the clinic in a tuktuk with a reported fractured leg. An X-ray subsequently verified a displaced fracture of the upper third of the tibia and fibula bones. I was initially informed that the leg had been smeared with turmeric with an improvised splint inadequately supporting the limb.

The man (a rubbish collector) had been hit by a car and had been told by people in his community that if he went to a hospital, he would have his leg amputated. Fortunately, this was not the case, and with the help of the outreach staff, he did subsequently receive the necessary surgery and welfare support.

One student I spoke to who was volunteering in the clinic said that children came in daily for wound cleaning and dressing. Many children also had toothache; however, there were not enough dentists for them to be seen. They were given a toothbrush and toothpaste, with some lessons on how to brush their teeth. The children were excited to see a short YouTube video and then try it themselves.

The student felt that the work at the clinic really made a difference, as the children didn't have any other opportunity to receive medical treatment. Therefore, it was a very rewarding month for her – both professionally and personally. She highly recommends the project and hopes to return.

What to expect at a Fijian hospital

At a Fijian hospital, expect to see skin infections, dog bites, fish bites, TB, stroke, heart disease, diabetes (previously undiagnosed), and hypertension, which has been untreated.

You may also witness many things rarely seen in developed countries, such as scabies and mumps. There can also be an enormous number of illnesses relating to Non-Communicable Diseases (NCDs).

Students are kept busy and can assist with injections, dressings, taking blood and conducting immunisations. Most students find it easy to adapt, and the staff are helpful and grateful.

A medical student at the more remote Savusavu Hospital reported more challenges, however, saying that there were 'some upsetting moments, but that was to be expected, and I guess it's part and parcel of working in a hospital in a less developed part of the world'.

Other feedback that we have received from medical students doing their elective in a Fijian hospital includes:

- 'I'm learning a lot and seeing lots of interesting cases. Everyone is very friendly and welcoming.'
- 'Everyone is super nice, which makes it very easy to settle in quickly. The medicine has been really interesting too!'
- 'The staff are treating me like family, and I am loving the whole experience.'

A Religion and Health Case Study – As told by one of our students: 'I was in the Emergency Department, when a 24-year-old first-time mum, 30 weeks pregnant, came in saying she was pre-ictal, and she felt the onset of a seizure about to happen. Naturally, it evoked concern in the medical team, who admitted the patient into a waiting bay to monitor both mother and child. I started helping the doctors cannulate and prepare the medication (first line was based on what was available, rather than what was best or least teratogenic); however, our progress in preparations was somewhat disturbed by the midwife who stood by the patient's side and prayed that the "daemons inside her left her alone".

'I was shocked to see a *medical professional* delaying things in such a way, and it showed me just how deeply religion runs in the community. It was not the only case that was left, temporarily at least, "in the hands of God". Luckily, this patient was cannulated and given diazepam as soon as the seizure started, and both she and her child were discharged the same day without any concerns.'

What to expect at a Sri Lankan hospital

Students have reported having a great time in Sri Lanka, and they often do a placement at the maternity hospital (or at the general hospital where they observe neurosurgery or oncology surgery) in the mornings and volunteer at local schools, orphanages or aged-care facilities in the afternoon.

What to expect at a Tongan hospital

A medical elective student spent two weeks at the main hospital, saying, 'I spent time in operating theatres, ICU, obstetrics and paediatrics. I could rotate around to whichever ward I wanted to be in, and the managers were very accommodating. I saw many surgeries I would not have otherwise been able to see at home.

'On the first day, I saw my first Caesarean section. My eyes welled up with tears at witnessing the beauty of new life being born into the world. While experiencing some of the most incredible moments of my time so far in Tonga, I also experienced some of the most difficult. Watching a baby struggle for life in ICU, partially as a result of lack of resources, compelled me to ask lots of questions, which I am thankful for.'

What to expect at a Tanzanian hospital

A student on placement in Tanzania felt that the outpatient department of the hospital was most interesting, as this was where patients attended with an astonishing array of problems ranging from everyday URTIs to facial lacerations from knife attacks, trauma, traumatic brain injuries, hypertensive crisis, hydrocephalus, renal failure, and heart failure.

There were also many dehydrated children with gastrointestinal infections. Performing small procedures such as suturing and wound care was another area where she was able to assist. Confidentiality and privacy do not seem to be a consideration in Tanzanian hospitals; however, the patients seemed respectful to one another.

Working with limited resources

Medical students are always amazed at how the local staff do an incredible job with the limited resources that they have available.

One student with a particular interest in surgery was able to see how different it was operating without the same resources used in hospitals in his home country (i.e. the use of spinal blocks instead of general anaesthetic for major operations).

A doctor volunteering in Cambodia said, 'I was frustrated somewhat by not being able to use imaging and blood tests that we regard as routine, mainly due to expense. So, for me it meant remembering basic physical examination from my early training, then a trial of treatment chosen on availability in the pharmacy, and then early review for the benefit of both patient and doctor.'

Equipment could also be second-hand, donated and/or very old. Simple supplies that we take for granted, such as dressing and tape, are used very frugally. Even pain relief medication may be administered only when absolutely needed. Oxygen saturation metres (pulse oximeter) seem to be in short supply everywhere.

Another student based in an emergency department recommended bringing a medical textbook for guidance, as there were a number of incidences in the busy ED where doctors were unsure of management.

There might also be a lack of education on how to manage equipment and supplies. Sometimes the staff have not sorted through what they have, and so if you go in *search* for specific items, you may actually find them if you look hard enough. The staff would also benefit from someone going there to assist with sorting through their supplies, setting up a storage system and educating them on how to use and maintain the equipment.

What the hospitals can lack

Generally, the hospitals in developing countries are quite overwhelming for those who haven't travelled to such countries.

Sometimes in the emergency department, the resuscitation beds are lucky to have oxygen, a pulse oximeter, blood pressure cuff and an old paddle defibrillator.

Likewise, the maternity ward can usually just be lined with beds holding both mother and neonate, as well as nearby beds with labouring women. The sterile gloves can even be found drying on a piece of string near the procedure room. A rare find of a sink with an old cake of soap can be amusing, as is the sign above it saying 'dry hands with own hanky'.

Many clinics and hospitals offer limited privacy for the patients. The consultation rooms may be an open space with zero confidentiality and could even have monkeys skipping overhead on the walls! An outpatient clinic could have doctors lined up side-by-side at a desk, and the patients sitting or standing opposite them to disclose their presenting complaint.

Despite what some hospitals might lack, life continues with its usual mix of tragedy and delight. You may ponder about the range of emotions seen and sometimes experienced during the course of a working day. One minute you could be moved to tears seeing a small girl with severe head trauma as a result of coming off a motorbike not having worn a helmet.

In this scenario, which I witnessed, the girl was sent home, as the hospital couldn't do anything for her. A nurse said, 'Only God can help her.'

The next minute, you could witness the delight on the face of a young man finally able to go home after a long stay in hospital due to a severe leg injury sustained in a motorbike accident. 'I can walk!' he said, as he hobbled past on his way back into the real world.

How to get the most out of your placement

By building trust, asking questions and offering to help, the local staff gain confidence in your ability to deliver.

A student said, 'To ensure I got the most from the program, I actively got involved with anything I could. Asking questions, following doctors to the patient's bedside, picking up X-rays and CT scans and assessing/examining patients every chance I got.'

Sometimes it may be appropriate to look for opportunities in other departments. After you have settled in, you are usually able to visit other units and talk with the nurses and doctors there and offer to help. Medical students should also gain some practical clinical skills beforehand so they can be more hands-on.

It is recommended that you find out in advance what your colleagues wear and then bring and wear the same (scrubs or white coat). Most visitors find that they are more readily accepted by staff and patients as part of the medical team while wearing the same gear, and this can help greatly in cementing a positive experience for you and also your colleagues.

Many students feel fortunate in being able to watch some amazing surgeries and sit in on clinical consultations with doctors. They find this incredibly rewarding and they learn so much.

Communicating at work

It can be challenging talking to a patient because of the language barrier. Learning some basic language in your country of choice will make life a little easier while working overseas; however, the nurses and doctors usually speak English.

The experience will put your communication skills to the test by relying on non-verbal cues and minimal English to assess and determine differential diagnosis. From working in the hospitals, it shouldn't take you long to pick up a few foreign words – knowing the appropriate words for 'pain' and 'breath' are probably the most helpful and beneficial to patient assessment.

Doctors and nurses often communicate with patients in their native language. However, in some countries the doctors often communicate with each other and do patient handovers in English. All medical records are mainly written in English.

A student in Nepal reported, 'Even though I could not speak the language, the power of non-verbal communication became evident. Although I found it difficult at first, I did not realise how much I could rely on this to see patients, especially those with anxiety – body language, a simple smile, a reassuring touch. This worked both ways. They were just always so appreciative of the treatment and bowed their heads to say thank you. To see their smiles as they left was extremely rewarding and made me grateful for such an experience. I still remember my first days when I found the language barrier difficult to treat patients. When I jumped this hurdle, I started to enjoy it, and I felt that I was really helping people. Their smiles were enough for me to understand that they really appreciated my work.'

What the supervisors are like

I stress the importance of developing friendships and building rapport with all of the staff. Many students have reported that socialising with doctors outside the hospital environment made their visit so much more interesting.

Students have also said that their supervisors were really helpful, extremely nice, happy to teach and very keen to share their knowledge and experience. Many students are also inspired by the staff's level of commitment to the job and their patients.

Fijians, in particular, are always friendly, and staff may even share their food at lunch.

Many students report that in Tanzania, in spite of the enormous difficulties that staff encountered on a daily basis, they always smiled. The patients, likewise, seemed to be very resilient and never seemed to complain no matter how long they had to wait to be seen. One mother displayed strong emotional resilience when one of her twins had died of birth asphyxia.

Students find working with the team in Cambodia to be such a pleasure. They feel really welcomed, and the staff often take them under their wings while exchanging stories about their lives in Battambang and at home.

Although undergraduate medical education is now well established in Nepal, graduate education programs have only recently been established. Most of the doctors are trained in countries other than Nepal, and they bring a broad and varied range of experience to clinical practice.

Wherever you carry out your elective, you will be sure to experience a myriad of personalities, and this is best dealt with by adopting a positive attitude an ongoing willingness to help in any way you can.

CHAPTER 7

WHEN THINGS GO WRONG ...

#shithappens

It's only natural that you might encounter some minor mishaps on your elective overseas, or there could be more dramatic events, such as an earthquake! Here are some suggestions on what to do if disaster strikes, or if there are daily 'issues' to overcome.

General issues that *can* arise

A frequent issue is that most of the local staff don't seem to know that the student is commencing their program. The Medical Superintendent or head matron is certainly aware; however, the message does not always filter down from the top through to the supervisor. Or maybe the supervisor is on leave or has just returned from leave, and they are still catching up on other important issues. Don't be concerned, and don't think that you are not welcome. Definitely don't take it personally – they simply have a lot on their plate.

A student once mentioned that they didn't think they were

expected in the hospital, as there was little direction given on arrival, and they were left on their own to choose where to work each day. They were fine with this because they could explore different wards. Therefore, don't be surprised or upset if this happens. Simply take the opportunity to use your initiative and put your communication skills into practice.

Another issue is that staff don't seem to have much work for you to do. This is common in your first few days and happens because they are not always familiar with your background, training and motivations. This is where communication and your attitude are key. Continue to show enthusiasm, ask questions, offer to help, and then keep offering to help with specific tasks (no matter how small or trivial). You will gain confidence in yourself and build the staff's trust as you complete more tasks and demonstrate that you are a valuable member of the team.

As I have previously mentioned, language can be a challenge. I recommend learning key words and medical terms of the country that you are visiting. The staff and patients will appreciate your efforts. If you feel that you are being excluded and too few staff speak English, it may be beneficial to raise your concerns with another staff member. You can also seek out local medical students and junior doctors because they will be more fluent in English. Many issues are fixable if you speak up (just remember to be polite, professional and respectful during the discussion).

One of our students in Tanzania was feeling a bit lost and useless at first, and the language barrier made it difficult for her to carry out what she wanted to do. However, her response was, 'I'm definitely sticking at it as it's been such an eye-opening and incredible experience so far, and I know it will get easier with time.' Like her, most students find that things seem to get easier as the days fly by, and they just persist with it.

It is also usually fine to move into other departments if you feel overwhelmed in a particular one or can see how you can assist better in another – the hospitals always seem to be fairly flexible. Just relax and enjoy the experience and do whatever you can to assist.

More concerning issues can include ill-health. Despite taking great care with hygiene, drinking bottled water and eating carefully prepared well-cooked foods, you may succumb to an upset stomach. Hopefully it will pass with some medication from your first aid kit and a day or two of rest. Don't hesitate to contact your travel insurer (via their 24/7 hotline) to discuss any issues that may have potential to develop into something more serious. Also note that you can buy meds over the counter in many countries where you may need a prescription in Australia, New Zealand, Canada, the USA, or the UK.

Bag Snatching – Petty theft and pickpockets are unfortunately a common occurrence anywhere in the world. We therefore recommend that you don't wear or take any expensive jewellery or valuables. Even though you are living and working in the country, you will still be viewed as a tourist. You may be a student; however, you will be considered wealthy by local standards and therefore become a target.

I have travelled extensively around the world as a solo female. I gain peace of mind by wearing a money belt under my clothes to carry my passport, credit card, cash and any valuable documents. Therefore, if someone wants to wrestle for my daypack or handbag, they are welcome to take it. Everything is replaceable (and probably covered by travel insurance); however, your life and your safety are non-negotiable – so don't risk it.

If you are subject to crime, ask your hosts to help you visit the police station to file a report and then claim on your travel insurance. It can be traumatic and unsettling, so I recommend talking to someone about it locally or phone a friend. Try not to let the incident spoil your day, your journey, or your faith in human beings.

Tanzania is generally considered safe for students and tourists and, although this is mostly the case, one student had the unfortunate experience of having her bag 'snatched' from her shoulder while walking from the hospital to the volunteer house one lunchtime. Having her camera and phone, along with a small amount of money, stolen was an unpleasant experience, but it was also a reminder about the need to exercise a reasonable degree of caution. Visiting the Moshi police station was not a highlight of the trip; however, she certainly didn't let it define the rest of her experience in such a wondrous country. She made a claim on her travel insurance for the stolen items, replaced them and continued to build new friends and fond memories of Tanzania.

Bed Bugs – I have heard of a couple of instances of bed bugs in Fiji, and this is not due to a lack of hygiene at the accommodation. Bed bugs are incredibly common (unfortunately) and often travel in someone's luggage. Bugs can live for months without food, thus making them ready stowaways and squatters. They don't pose any serious medical risk; however, the stubborn parasites can leave itchy and unsightly bites. An affected room will usually require professional help to exterminate via fumigation and sealing off the area for a day or two.

Natural Disasters – Natural disasters happen randomly and unexpectedly. There frequently seems to be a cyclone, flood, drought, earthquake, bushfire, civil unrest, terrorism or some other event somewhere in the world (and even in your own backyard).

I had arranged for some medical students to do their elective in Nepal. A major earthquake struck while they were there in April 2015. Luckily, the students were safe and well cared for.

However, with many earthquakes, there is the risk of aftershocks, and gaining access to clean water, food and power becomes stretched. Infrastructure (power, transport, buildings and hospitals) may be compromised. After discussing the situation with the students' university and travel insurer, they were evacuated from Kathmandu on a Royal Australian Air Force jet to Bangkok (they were fortunately offered seats on the second RAAF flight that departed a few days after the earthquake).

One of our students was in Fiji when Cyclone Winston hit in February 2016. She was told to buy emergency supplies, and then, as the weather got wilder, she climbed into the bathtub with plenty of bedding. She remained safe and comfortable while reading her book and snacking on chocolate biscuits as the cyclone raged around her.

In summary, if something goes wrong or doesn't feel right, approach any or all of the following people:

- Your local hosts at your accommodation or at work. They will have knowledge and advice on how to resolve most issues.
- Your travel insurer (particularly for health and safety advice and any incidences, loss or change of travel plans that may result in a claim).
- Your student medical indemnity provider (particularly if there is an issue with a patient, or an incident or an accident at work).
- Your university co-ordinator, your parents, your elective arranger.
- Embassy of your home country.

We have heard many students advise their friends to 'tell DocTours if you have an issue, as they will endeavour to find a solution', and it is important to us to know that you can count on our help, as we are always able to assist you in any way you might need.

CHAPTER 8

AFTER HOURS

#travelstories

Let's now discuss the variety of adventures you can have 'after hours' – and I have plenty of suggestions for you in this chapter to really take your trip to the next level. Whether you spend a night in a Buddhist monastery, trek iconic mountains, visit traditional villages or embark on a jungle safari, there is much to see and do outside the hospital during your travels.

An example of a unique experience that you would only get overseas

One of my most memorable experiences was on a trip to Nepal. And you too can enjoy this adventure if you head there, because a trip to Nepal would be incomplete if you didn't experience the Royal Chitwan National Park.

Leaving home at 4.45 am (yes, it will be dark and very cold), catch a 'tourist' bus from Kathmandu to Sauraha (Chitwan). It is great to get away from the chaos and dust of Kathmandu and take in some breathtaking scenery on the outskirts of town.

Traffic in developing countries is always a bit hair-raising, and the drive to Chitwan is no different. Crowded roads, speeding, and musical horns all play their part as traffic hurtles through the mountains.

The drive was spectacular as we followed the vertiginous mountains and emerging clear, blue waters of the Rapti River valley southbound. The driver stopped every two hours for a reviver, and some of the passengers visited the roadside kiosks to sample a local curry or to buy oranges. There was also an optional visit to the adjacent small tin sheds with a hole in the ground, which offered limited privacy for doing 'your business'.

At Chitwan there is a popular hotel called the Eden Resort, which provides great food, accommodation and a two-day program for tourists. The park's activities include guided jungle walks and a canoe ride through the early morning mist. These are flat-bottomed timber canoes without a keel to help stabilise the vessel.

Thankfully, they provided us with little green life jackets before we proceeded through several series of rapids over the freezing water. The birdlife was amazing, and we saw many deer, monkeys and peacocks. If your canoe becomes grounded mid-stream, the captain won't hesitate to leap barefoot into the water to push the canoe forward. 'Are there crocodiles?' Yes. 'Freezing water?' Definitely.

The elephant safari provides an opportunity to explore the jungle from the height and relative safety of an elephant's back. The beauty being that you are able to ride within metres of animals such as rhinos and white-spotted deer without them knowing. The jeep safari offers more opportunity to spot rhinos, crocodiles, white-spotted deer, wild boar, kingfisher birds, monkeys, and much more; however, a tiger can prove to be elusive. Finally, I recommend that you embark on a safari on foot (no jeeps) with the only 'protection' being a bamboo stick. Good luck fending off a tiger with that!

Chitwan is a touristy area and there is some fantastic souvenir shopping in the town. They also have an evening cultural show with music, and singers and dancers dressed in local costumes. The performance is really enjoyable and worthwhile attending.

Some students camped out in Dolalghat for two days, which is a fishermen's village that was largely destroyed in the 2015 earthquake. The locals rebuilt and completed the building of new homes by using materials donated by Rotary Northbridge. It was so interesting to learn about practical issues when trying to rebuild homes in Nepal. The nearest road ended far from the village and the locals carried steel panels up 100 metres of mountain terrain. A village may be a ten-hour walk to the nearest road, and so it is difficult to imagine someone walking that distance while unwell and needing hospitalisation.

It was truly amazing (and very challenging) camping out in a village with people so far removed from Western tourism and Western culture. They cooked dinner in the evening, and despite the humble conditions, the food was delicious.

Joining in the celebrations for the festival of Diwali (basically Christmas for Hindus) was also a highlight. Buildings were covered in (Christmas) lights, and children went door to door singing with candles. In the evenings, everyone enjoyed a feast! The party went for a week, and everyone dressed up in full Nepali kit and ventured into Thamel for the rituals.

There are some very cool temples in Kathmandu, and Pokhara is a very popular and beautiful town by Lake Fewa. Visiting nearby Sarangkot for sunrise and seeing the astonishing Annapurna Ranges for the first time at dawn is an experience that many people never forget! Paragliding at sunrise provides amazing views over Pokhara and Fewa Lake.

There are short two-day treks in Pokhara to the 'Australia Camp'. The view from the guesthouse in the Australia Camp of the Annapurna Ranges, including Fish Tail, is breathtaking. Watching the sunrise on the rooftop and seeing the clouds clear to show these majestic white peaks is a magical experience that many people highly recommend.

Get involved in community projects

A community project may take place at a remote school, or at a hostel for old people or the disabled, and it is an opportunity to provide basic health care and lessons on health and hygiene to the local people.

Nepal – Many students feel very fortunate to visit government schools in Nepal where the children can't afford to seek medical attention. The children, ranging from 5–15 years old, are given a dental hygiene kit, as well as a health check assessment. Most students really enjoy this program, as they can see that they make a difference among the community by providing health services. The kids are also great fun to be with.

I once travelled with a group of young medical students volunteering in Nepal. Visiting three schools in the Kathmandu Valley, we delivered classes to the local children about health care and good hygiene practice.

At the first school, we worked with a group of teenagers aged 15–18 years who were studying biology. The morning kicked off with a formal welcome and a cultural display of folk dancing in colourful national costume. One of our medical students then delivered demonstrations on good oral hygiene and how to carefully and correctly roll a condom onto a banana. We then organised ourselves into teams based on skill sets and set up our medical clinics in some of the classrooms. Males and females were split into different groups for discussions on mental and sexual health.

We took the children's vital signs and then sat down for one-on-one consults. Our goal was for the local teenage students to view the medical students as peers of a similar age and thus feel comfortable in talking to them about any issues of concern. Interestingly, dehydration seemed to be quite common and was manifesting itself in many ways. The day ended with the international basketball championships. It was a fantastic way to break down barriers through participating in sporting activities and learning about their cultural activities.

The next morning, our medical students visited a local school for 72 deaf children. Again, they demonstrated good health care to the children and then undertook mini-health checks. Their schoolteachers helped with interpretation and also arranged follow-ups, as well as providing ongoing health education for the students.

The next stop was a remote high school located in a very poor neighbourhood. By this stage, our med students were growing more confident in setting up a pop-up clinic and delivering basic health care to the Nepali children.

Fiji – The people of Fiji are known for their kindness and generosity, and there's no doubt, given the warm welcome guests receive. Visitors are often invited to people's villages, homes, weddings and religious ceremonies. The program is very appealing because students can work with doctors in the hospital and also on outreach programs with nurses providing and promoting health education in villages and schools.

Non-Communicable Diseases such as diabetes and heart disease are an increasing issue for the local community. The major risk factors are obesity, lack of exercise, eating the wrong food, smoking, and excessive drinking of alcohol and kava. The purpose of the outreach clinics is to tackle these issues.

The clinics are usually comprised of one doctor and two nurses – one nurse from the village (the only health care they have easy access to) and one from the hospital, which is a two-hour drive over rough ground.

Simple measurements (BMI, blood glucose and blood pressure) are used to ascertain the patients' general conditions, and prescriptions for medications are given out accordingly. Generally, the supply is quickly used up and patients at the end of the line only receive a prescription (interestingly, the nurses didn't think that the patients would actually acquire the medication).

While in the village, there was a nurse-led education session on diet, exercise, and the importance of medication compliance.

In Fiji, one in three adults have diabetes, and thus it is paramount that the health care given educates as well as treats specific problems. On many visits, we are continually surprised by how late some patients present with issues, often with BMs in the 30s, and many with diabetic foot sepsis.

Cambodia – Riding my bicycle down the river road towards the medical clinic, when I was on a more recent visit, the traffic was a weaving sea of mottos, bicycles, tuktuks and cars. There was an 'ordered chaos' where everyone seemed to know what the other was about to do – there was never any road rage and you rarely saw any collisions.

People were starting their day selling a variety of goods that ranged from one-litre bottles of petrol to fresh sugar cane juice. Children were scouring for rubbish that could be sold to the recyclers, and groups of happy, naked children played in the dirt or waved as I rode by. Mothers were sitting in the shade with babes on their knees, in front of ramshackle houses embellished by clothes hanging on fences to dry.

It was only 7.30 am, but I was a lather of perspiration when I finally arrived in the bougainvillea-laced laneway and parked my bike. Children called out 'hello' and smiled, or they ran up to hold my hand, looking up at me with their lovely dark-brown eyes and innocent faces.

The school I was visiting was an NGO (Non-Government

Organisation) in a slum area of Siem Reap, and it provided free education to the children in the surrounding area, and still does.

The Cambodian who founded the school realised that education was the only way out of the poverty cycle. As NGOs rely on sponsorship and donations, the classrooms are basic: a blackboard and a fan.

In addition to this clinic, there is a school and a restaurant that trains the locals in the hospitality industry. At lunchtime (or rather 'siesta'), we were able to sample the many varieties of dishes freshly prepared by the student chefs, along with tasty lime and mango juices.

When the weekend arrived, a dental student visited an orphanage in Battambang, where she gave the children oral hygiene lessons, with the head of the orphanage translating for her. She had brought toothbrushes, toothpaste, certificates and stickers with her, all donated by GlaxoSmithKline, and it was extremely fulfilling to watch the children perfect their techniques as they brushed their teeth. It was a wonderful end to a life-changing week.

Another student went to Cambodia for her elective and also took the opportunity to help teach English. She was feeling a bit apprehensive, as she wasn't sure how much she would remember about English grammar. Every day began with a school assembly in the courtyard. The students were lined up in rows of boys and rows of girls.

At the beginning of every class, the students would stand with their hands in prayer and say, 'Good morning teacher. How are you today?'

The teacher would then respond with, 'I'm fine, thank you, and how are you?'

The students then replied, 'I'm fine, thank you'. Then they waited to be told they could sit down.

She found it was a real delight working with the children who seemed happy and readily embraced her. The children really appreciated having volunteers help in their classes and they gladly accepted foreigners.

Tanzania – During their free time in Moshi, many students take the opportunity to volunteer in other areas – visiting an orphanage, a school, or helping with an environmental project. They also generally tour some of the smaller villages, visiting coffee and banana plantations, and they can cool off with a swim in a volcanic pond at the base of a spectacular waterfall.

Experiences after hours

You will find that there is much more to your visit than what you accomplish while 'at work'. Many students have reported of hosts going above and beyond what they could have ever expected, as well as having adventures that they thought were only a dream. Here's just a few 'after hours' activities to give you an idea of what is waiting for you …

Nepal – A student had a birthday during her first few days in Nepal, and her host family surprised her with a special dinner! They baked a chocolate and peanut cake, decorated it with candles, and they cooked delicious curries, chicken and rice. It was an incredible and memorable birthday, and she was incredibly grateful to them for making her feel so special.

On her last night in Nepal, she was invited to go to a 'dinner party' with her host family. They all dressed up and travelled by bus into Kathmandu. On arrival she was surprised that it was in fact a wedding that she was lucky enough to attend. There was so much amazing food, joyful entertainment, and happy, friendly guests – she couldn't wipe the smile off her face for days. She felt so lucky to be included in this occasion and could not thank the family enough for everything they had done over the past four weeks.

Cambodia – When relaxing after hours in Cambodia, it is easy to tap into the Wi-Fi network, enjoy an Angkor beer (at $1 a shot) and the amazing sunrise over Angkor Wat near Siem Reap. This is a stunning spectacle, and the more clandestine temples of Ta Prohm and Bayon are all definitely worth a visit.

The locals here are so welcoming and hospitable, always sharing their stories, food and laughter. The more adventurous try the local delicacy of fried crickets and mice, and they assured me that they both tasted delicious!

Everyone squeezes in some sightseeing. The highlights in Battambang include travelling on a motorbike with the local nurses to see the top of a mountain, watching a million bats come out of a cave at sunset, and riding the 'bamboo' train. Battambang completely captures the heart: the people, the food, and the peacefulness about the place.

Tonga – A nursing student landed in Fua'amotu International Airport alone and unsure of how she would find her way; however, she knew she was in for an unforgettable experience. Immediately after landing, Tongan hospitality was demonstrated by a stranger who invited her to their cousin's wedding the next day. The student believed that this would be a great way to settle into a new country.

The wedding invite led to being invited to church on Sunday morning, and a wedding feast that afternoon. She remarked that Tongan people sure knew how to feast! Suckling pigs, octopus, turtle and lobsters were among the delicacies prepared by the bride's family. Other highlights in Tonga include visiting neighbouring islands for snorkelling, swimming with the whales, great food and beautiful beaches.

Fiji – Take some time to explore and have a holiday when you're in Fiji! The opportunities for either relaxation or adventure are endless. And why not learn more about Fiji by saying 'yes' to the different tasks and experiences that come your way. Keep the phone numbers of a couple of drivers to get you around locally. The drivers are generally friendly and make you feel safe. For the ladies, wear long, light skirts – particularly when visiting remote areas.

Tanzania – An African safari was one of the most amazing experiences of my life when I was there. Moshi is a beautiful town, and the people, especially children, are really friendly. You will no doubt meet many fantastic people, and also have the chance to eat all the local food and discover the Moshi nightlife. Going on safari and climbing Mount Kilimanjaro are highlights of visiting Tanzania. Zanzibar is also beautiful and well worth the visit, especially to help you wind down after some eye-opening experiences.

AFRICA

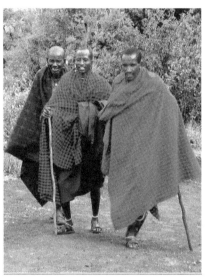

The Maasai are an ethnic group inhabiting northern, central and southern Kenya and northern Tanzania.

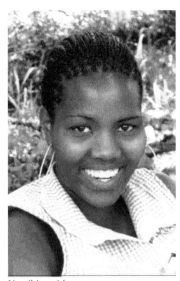

Namibian girl

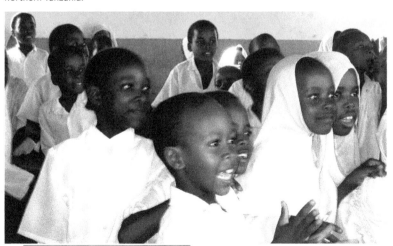

School in Africa

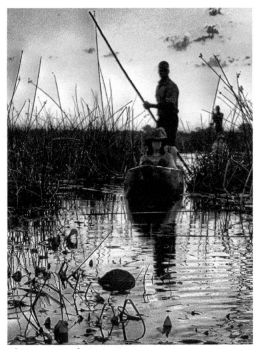

African water safari

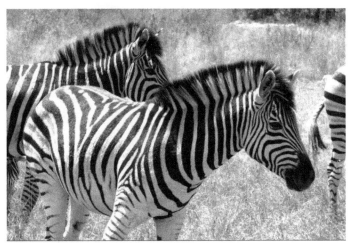

Zebras are one of Africa's best-known animals, and Namibia is home to two of the four species that roam the plains of Africa in large numbers.

CAMBODIA

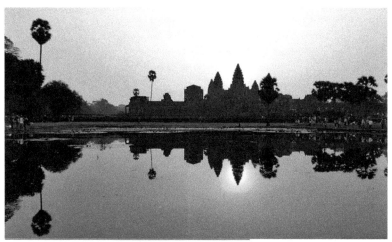

Temples of Angkor, in Cambodia.

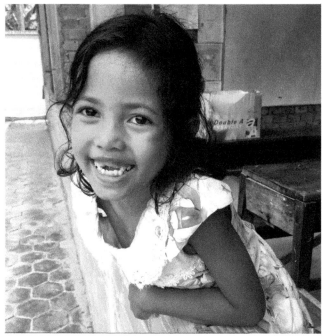

A Cambodian school girl.

SRI LANKA

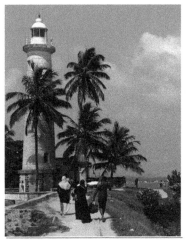

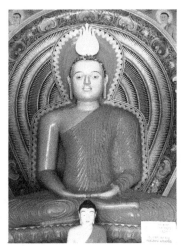

Galle is a city on the southwest coast of Sri Lanka. It's known for Galle Fort, the

Sri Lanka temple.

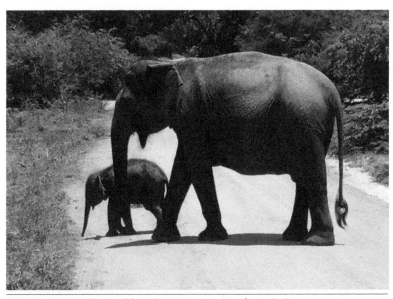

Sri Lanka has incredible wildlife walking around and a safari is the best way to see elephants.

NEPAL

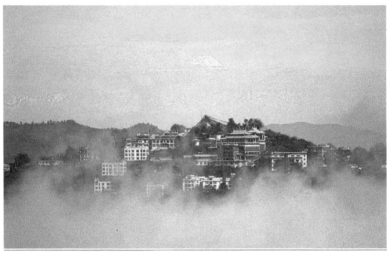

Namo Buddha is one of the most sacred Buddhist pilgrimage sites in Nepal. It is about two hours' drive from the city of Kathmandu

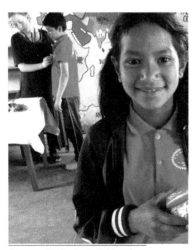

Community Projects in Nepal

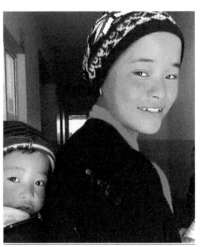

A Nepalese mum, carrying her child.

TONGA

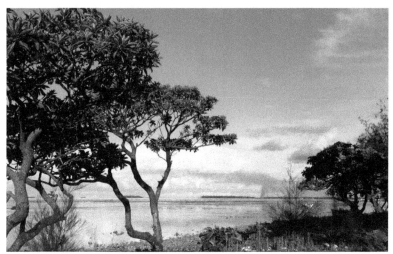

A beach in Tonga

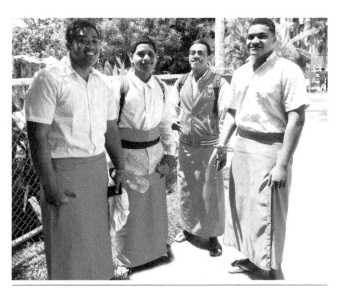

Tongan men wear a tupenu, a cloth that is wrapped around the waist. On formal occasions a ta'ovala, a woven mat, is worn over the tupenu. It is wrapped around the waist and secured with a kafa rope.

FIJI

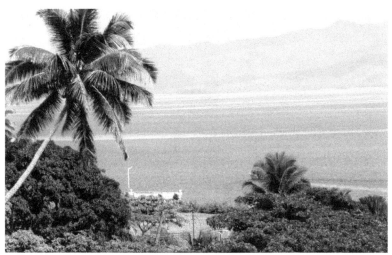

Blue sea in Fiji

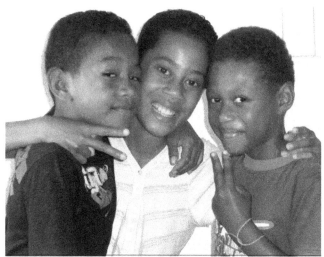

Fiji kids.

ECUADOR

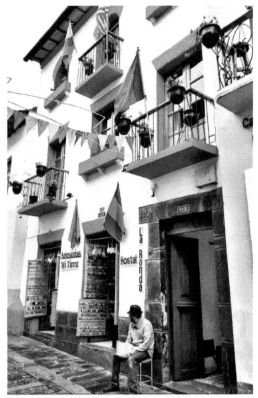

A hostel in Guayaquil, Ecuador.

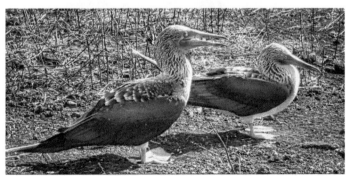

The famous Blue-Footed Booby, in Galapagos Islands.

SECTION THREE

||||||||||||||||||||||||||||||||||||||||||||||||||||||||||||||||||||||||||||||||||||||||||||||||||||||||||||||

Review, Reflect and Report on Your Elective Journey

Many students consider their international elective to have been the most enlightening, humbling and fascinating learning experience of their lives. They expected to be challenged; however, the challenges came from where they least expected and they felt they had developed both professionally and personally.

Their journey and the myriad experiences have helped define and shape their future career paths, as well as their motivation for medicine. It has also given them a greater awareness of global health and deepened their desire to travel and explore our wonderful world more.

CHAPTER 9

REVIEW AND REFLECT ON YOUR ELECTIVE

#keepexploring

Coming home is usually with mixed feelings. You may be looking forward to your own bed, your favourite food, and seeing familiar faces. On the other hand, saying goodbye to new friends and marking the end of an incredible journey can be sad. So, take some time to reflect on your amazing, life-changing journey.

I frequently receive accounts from our students, and it is always quite heart-warming to read about each of their special and unique experiences. One young student said, 'The past four weeks has been an amazing, eye-opening and unique experience whereby I have gained an enormous appreciation for the health care system we have back home.'

It is very rare to hear of anyone regretting their decision to travel, and virtually all students report that they are so glad that they went overseas for their elective.

Another student confessed that she had signed up for her elective not knowing anyone, and she realised afterwards that she'd be missing weeks of compulsory medical classes, which would take months to catch up on. However, she believed that it was 100 percent worth it for the array of people she met. Even though there were totally different personalities found on foreign soil, people somehow gelled. The medical experience, the adventure and, most importantly, the perspective gave her the motivation to get through the last part of her medical degree and made it all worthwhile.

A young nurse I spoke with had been thinking about volunteering in a totally different environment and taking a break from her usual mundane nursing work. Before she knew it, she found herself on the road to discovery, describing it as an 'unforgettable experience of a lifetime'.

A junior doctor told me that her friends queried why she would spend precious holidays during her intern year on a medical volunteering trip. She wasn't completely convinced of her own decision until she walked out of the foreign airport into the bustling, dusty streets of a different world. At that moment, she knew she was in for a once-in-a-lifetime experience.

A recent graduate reflected: 'Nepal is a country that can take your breath away. Not only will the beautiful Himalayas leave you breathless, but so will the scenes of poverty and underdevelopment. I feel lucky to have experienced a fortnight of medical volunteering in this amazing country that is such a different world to my own.'

A final year medical elective student in Fiji described the impact: 'I have become passionate about the idea of working abroad and hope to be able to spend more time abroad throughout my career. I really enjoyed being able to see the different health care provisions, as well as how different cultures regard their own health. I left Fiji with new friends and a renewed perspective that I'm sure will lure me back to the Pacific region. I learnt so much and gained so much experience in such a short space of time. I have grown both personally and professionally and couldn't have asked for a more hospitable, warm and welcoming group of people who made my elective even more enjoyable!'

Final reflections

Your learning and development experiences may emerge in many ways, and the key take-aways can be summarised in four main areas:

1. **Clinical** – students gain an insight into working in a lower income setting and are exposed to conditions and treatments not common at home. Their confidence and competence often grow while taking part in routine clinical practices.

2. **Cultural** – seeing firsthand how different social attitudes to health (particularly traditional medicine) can influence health outcomes, both positively and negatively.

3. **Personal** – many become passionate about the idea of working abroad and hope to be able to spend more time in different countries. They leave their placement with new friends and a renewed perspective with good intentions to return in the future.

4. **Medical School** – their journey is a reminder as to why they wanted to do medicine and provides renewed enthusiasm towards their study.

Reflecting on the homestay experience

Most people enjoy the homestay experience and appreciate the extra level of attention and support given by people who genuinely care. Hosts often do everything possible to make the volunteering experience one to remember. They make you feel part of their family, welcoming you into their home and treating you like one of their own.

They incorporate cultural experiences and festivals into your schedule so that you have a unique, special involvement in the local way of life. Home cooking is often a highlight, and host families provide traditional meals (usually with a moderated level of spice), as well as support and guidance throughout the program.

Many students feel very fortunate to enjoy the warmth and support of family accommodation. They also have the opportunity to meet many travellers from around the world and can share stories, tips and information. Staying with locals and living away from a large city can readily provide insights into what life is actually like for the local people. There is a lot of appreciation for the efforts that host families make to ensure that everyone's visit is an action-packed authentic experience.

Hosts often share stories of their history, culture, and current political situations, and they can provide multidimensional knowledge of the local community, its strengths, weaknesses and needs. Their social, interpersonal and professional skills place them in the privileged position of making a significant difference to the lives of many. And their ability to engage international volunteers from a variety of backgrounds is of enormous value, as they are usually well connected and understand the needs of the community.

Hospitality and friendliness offered by complete strangers is often beyond description, and well-chosen hosts have a natural ability of making guests feel welcome and comfortable. They may offer shelter to visitors; however, more importantly, they offer a home!

One student recounted, 'We quickly came to realise the warmth and generosity of the Nepali people that is often spoken about, which was embodied by this lovely couple. We were given an affectionate welcome by our host who garlanded us with the traditional golden scarf and topped it off with a hug.'

Another said, 'I was hosted by a local family who are the most beautiful people. You couldn't ask for a better platform for exploring a new country.'

What previous students and volunteers have learnt

Returning students regale a plethora of suggestions to prospective medical students looking to complete their elective in a developing country. Here are some of the more insightful ones for the countries of choice.

Take the opportunity (where possible) to do school health checks and village health camps as well as gaining experience in the hospital. This gives you a great opportunity to use your history-taking and examination skills. You have more responsibility and sovereignty when it comes to seeing and managing your own patients. A common theme from many students who suggested this was that some of the most valuable learning experiences are outside of the hospital, so many students appreciated the flexibility to come and go.

Many students had a wonderful time with people that they met throughout the trip. They noted that their eyes were opened to a whole new world in general and a new health care system. With the continuous support and encouragement from staff, they began to handle many duties and discuss a variety of diagnoses, care plans and treatments with local medical staff.

Some students reported that their experience shaped their career decisions and made a huge impact on their drive and passion for medicine. Their time overseas was an eye-opener and verified their dedication to their career path. By being able to learn from local specialists and listen to the problems that local people faced in a developing country, this provided inspiration. Despite gender inequality still being quite a profound issue in developing countries, it is great to see that there is so much influence coming from international groups, such as Rotary, in improving global health.

Other students were driven to change their career paths. Young nurses and physiotherapists have told me that they felt that their time overseas was an important aspect of proving to themselves, as well as others, that medicine (and to become a doctor) was where they wanted to dedicate their life.

There are bound to be many patient cases that you will see overseas that you just won't experience in Australia, New Zealand, Canada, the USA, or the UK. Some students who were based in orthopaedics generally worked six days per week and saw a good mix of clinic and surgical patients. However, they also ventured in and out of emergency, where they saw the odd case such as assisting with the resuscitation of a two-year-old child that had been stung by killer bees and who had subsequently gone into disseminated intravascular coagulation.

The most important recommendation is to just show up with an open mind and go with the flow. Local staff will do things their own way and at their own pace. This can be frustrating at times, so having patience helps.

Many students expected to be challenged; however, the challenges they found came from where they least expected. Therefore, be ready and willing to adapt and then treat it as a *learning experience* – both professionally and personally.

Many students' first impressions of a developing country are often described as 'culture shock', and that's coming from students who are usually well travelled and have experienced many parts of Southeast Asia. I expected to see extreme poverty and a lack of resources. However, it is often a surprise to see how resourceful these countries are with their medical personnel and supplies.

When students return home and sit down to study or start work in a modern hospital or clinic, they feel so fortunate to have had the opportunity to work overseas. They usually hope that they can be as calm and easy-going as the people in these developing countries, who never seem to get flustered.

Your view of the world can also be challenged. The 'island time' followed in some countries, such as Fiji and Tonga, can take some getting used to, and this way of living permeates the hospital too.

The pace is slow, and the nurses' workloads are lightened some-what by the fact that families do most of the personal care for patients. After the initial shock and adjusting to their alternative ways of being, many students adapt and enjoy the slower pace. Even after returning home to our busy lives, many yearn for the slower, simpler lifestyle.

Comparisons

It is natural to compare a developing country's facilities with that of a developed country's hospitals. Whatever differences you discover, it is important to remain respectful. Some of the other challenges of the health care systems in a developing country include:

- Lack of infrastructure – electricity supply can be unreliable, and there is a lack of government services for garbage collection, sewerage and clean water. Indoor air pollution is also an issue due to internal fires being used to cook meals in the home.
- Transportation – the main form of transport is via foot, bicycle or motorbike, and roads can be in poor condition. The injured may walk for two to three days to get to a hospital. Patients therefore want to have everything treated on a single visit to the doctor. Patients may discharge themselves prematurely and then need to re-present shortly after.
- Caste system – this is not recognised by their government; however, it is still a challenge in some countries.
- Faith healers – there are still people who consult their local priest when they are ill.
- Gender roles – females seem to do their fair share of the 'dirty work' and the heavy lifting on construction sites. They often return to work very quickly after giving birth, and prolapsed uterus seems to be quite common in many countries. In addition, during menstruation, some women in remote areas are not allowed in the home and can't prepare food,

and they sleep outside with the farm animals. This seems to manifest itself into infectious diseases, including brucellosis, respiratory, typhoid, UTIs, and maternal complications.

- Health insurance does not exist – a patient's family often needs to pay for materials and medical supplies (often prior to receiving any treatment).
- The patient's family also performs the personal care required for the patient (bathing, feeding and provision of food).
- Pharmacy – many pharmacists are not well trained and there is a lack of regulation, which results in the ongoing risk of counterfeit drugs. Medications are often obtained over the counter (without a prescription), and compliance may be poor.

A student once told me that when she was working in a hospital in Nepal, she realised that the average age of patients was about 30 years younger than the average Australian patient. Their presentations and diseases were also different to what she was used to – typhoid fever, TB, hepatitis, paratyphoid fever, impalement by a buffalo, and then more typhoid fever.

And it's not just the patients and their conditions that are different to what you might experience at home.

Many students are surprised to find that there is Wi-Fi available and everyone has a mobile phone; however, there may be frequent power cuts. And not only that, but hospitals may reuse needles and there is no sanitary running water. It is also not uncommon to hear of enduring cold showers, as the hot water systems may only work intermittently, and the 'flushed' toilet might require manual flushing with buckets of water.

Life can be frustrating while cold-showering in someone's bathroom, when the lights go out, the water trickles to a stop, and the torch battery dies while you are still caked in shampoo and soap. However, we remind ourselves that this is not for a lifetime, as it is for others.

Returning in future

Students returning from their international elective often tell me how the whole experience has left them wanting to do more, and they can see themselves doing more volunteering in the future, as they have seen how providing health care can make a real change to people's lives.

They return home with a large number of unforgettable experiences that have been accumulated in a relatively short time overseas. Almost always they state that they would love to have stayed for longer and will endeavour to return there in the future.

They express gratitude due to the success of the entire trip, and they look forward to exploring more international destinations. Many interns and registrars have even asked DocTours to arrange international placements for them so that they too can make further impacts on others in need in developing countries, as well as have the experience of a lifetime.

A student said, 'It has been an incredible experience to see how the health care system operates in a developing country. Compared with an Australian metropolitan tertiary hospital with fully equipped health care services, this trip has been an eye-opener to how a remote hospital in a developing country functions with so little resources.'

Another student wrote: 'Just wanted to write and thank you for arranging my placement in Battambang. I had a wonderful time on placement and do hope to return in the future. The experience was so fulfilling (as I expected it to be), and it does make coming home difficult. Thank you for always being contactable and for assisting me throughout.'

CHAPTER 10

REFLECT ON YOUR JOURNEY AND THE IMPACT ON LOCALS

#wanderingsoul

You may have been feeling excited or nervous before embarking on your international elective. You may have been worried about meeting the expectations of local staff, or thinking about whether the staff would meet your expectations. Whatever the case, it is worthwhile considering what impact you (and others) may have on the local people and the local staff. How did they respond to you during your time there, and what might you do differently the next time you walk into a new environment?

Your impact on locals

Many of our students are quite humble and do not notice the extent of their personal contribution or understand the huge benefit of what they do. Some people question the value of medical missions and 'voluntourism'; however, the benefits emerge on many fronts.

First and foremost, there are warm smiles and words of

gratitude received from patients. Volunteers also share their knowledge, skills and experience with the local staff, and the tangible donations of medical supplies and equipment are frequently made to continue the good work. Most importantly, volunteers demonstrate to the local people that someone cares about them – by just being there.

There is often a larger impact made when taking part in the community outreach programs in remote areas. These remote areas struggle to get access to resources and the skills of a medical professional; therefore, they always seem to be very appreciative of the visiting students.

Running a health clinic for community members and visiting a government school where the children could not afford to attend regular health check-ups is an incredible experience. This assists in breaking down international barriers and helps local people become more familiar with modern medicine. Performing public health checks is a great way to get involved, contribute to the local village, and students feel that they are truly able to make a difference.

Many nurses have volunteered in remote clinics and delivered training for staff on the 'Days for Girls' (DfG) menstruation kits. They often walk away with a huge respect for the people that continue to face challenges in their daily existence. The local people have so little, and yet they are generous, kind, caring and positive, and they are especially grateful for assistance in supporting their dignity. Local people are always keen to attend a clinic when there is a foreign doctor visiting.

When interacting with local kids on a daily basis as you walk to work, they soon recognise you, wave hello and call your name. Students always seem to be rewarded with gratitude, lots of smiles, and kind hospitality of a local coffee or tea. Occasionally, there is a gift of a traditional scarf or locally made craft. The people living in these developing countries teach us more about resilience and strength than what we teach them. There are frequent invitations to return to visit them, and many students sincerely hope they can.

One student reported that without exception, the Khmer people that he looked after were profusely grateful for the attention. They expressed this with a broad smile, a bow of the head with hands in the prayer position, while repeatedly saying 'or-koon'.

Volunteers have even visited rural schools to donate clothing and equipment. The donation of a computer was an invaluable gift, as the solution to building a better life lies in *education* and good health. The exposure to just one shared computer can make a world of difference. What is always really touching is the appreciation received from the schools. They typically hold a ceremony and present volunteers with a small gift and provide lunch. It makes you realise just how significant a small contribution can be.

A group of medical students were once overwhelmed when they completed the health checks at the school for deaf children on a cold winter day in Nepal. As they left, the deaf children sang to them, 'You have made our hearts warm'.

Many volunteers report that even after returning home, the memories of working overseas are vivid and stay with them forever. One remembers a ten-year-old boy who took his eight-year-old brother on his bicycle for several kilometres to be seen at the clinic. The younger brother had cut his foot on some metal a few days earlier and the wound had become infected. The boys were being cared for by their thirteen-year-old brother while their mother had gone to Thailand. Both boys were very dirty, so they were given clean T-shirts. After dressing the younger boy's foot, they rode off again down the laneway.

Visions of new mothers coming in to receive formula for their babies under the free formula program is another memorable experience. The mothers are too malnourished to support their babies with breast-feeding, and even with the formula, the baby's growth is well below the rates that you see in developed countries.

I once witnessed the gratitude and relief on the face of a young man who gave the volunteers a blessing that was normally given to royalty. They had cleaned his badly infected foot and dressed it. Even though he could barely walk, he had continued to work, as he had no other source of income. He was given some rice and sauce so that he could stop working for a day or two to rest his foot.

These images and memories are deeply touching, and many students return for another 'tour of duty'. The work that is being done by medical students and the local staff makes a difference to many lives, reversing the cycle of poverty and despair that these people would otherwise be trapped in.

Your impact on local doctors and nurses

There is enormous respect and admiration for many doctors and nurses in developing countries. They put in a huge effort every day for their critically ill patients, working extra hours and doing everything they can with the few resources that they have available. When power is lost several times during an operation, staff deal with it without complaint.

With the opportunity to see how the local staff assess and manage patients (heavily relying on non-verbal communication skills to do so), this helps you build essential skills such as adaptability, communication and teamwork, and it also assists you in developing as a health care professional. One of our students recommended that others should 'go with an open mind and heart, be prepared for culture shock, do what you can and have a wonderful experience'.

The most important thing a volunteer health care professional can do is provide a *sense of safety* and *comfort* for the local staff.

As visitors in their environment, it is a privilege and an honour to be welcomed and involved in their community. We all must remain kind and respectful of their culture and protocols while offering alternative treatments and options. We do not impose our ways onto the locals, expecting them to choose our ways over theirs. Creating change is difficult and takes time, so we proceed gently.

International volunteers and students are greatly appreciated

Students always seem to feel welcomed by both local staff and patients in international locations. Who would not appreciate an extra pair of hands from some energetic and enthusiastic students who are quick to learn?

Doctors in a hospital in Fiji have told me how grateful they are to have the extra support when it is busy. For example, a student can obtain specific medical supplies from the storeroom or pharmacy, and they can assist with taking histories, dressing wounds and carrying out many basic procedures to save time for the local staff. DocTours receives a lot of positive feedback from overseas clinics that reinforces the view that medical students and volunteers are well regarded and appreciated.

One of the supervising consultants in Fiji stated, 'I was very happy with the contribution, commitment and teamwork displayed. I found the volunteer's expertise in Scopes and scans very useful. Staff exposed her to areas such as oncology and working in a low-resource setting, which was appreciated by the volunteer doctor. The team appeared to have loved working with her and we'd appreciate it if you could convey this to her too. I personally believe it was a very worthwhile attachment.'

A clinic manager in Cambodia wrote to me: 'Thank you so much for your hard work, understanding and wonderful support in finding enthusiastic, skilful volunteers to assist at the clinic. How lovely it was to have the assistance, and all the staff were grateful for the enthusiasm, hard work and support. The doctors have been amazing with looking after our patients and also teaching our local doctor. They instantly became an important part of the team, and I feel quite sad that they have left. Thank you for recruiting such high calibre staff for us.'

CONCLUSION

Your journey through life will have many challenges and incredible experiences; however, your international medical elective should be one of the highlights. It is the opportunity to spend a month or two living and working in an international destination, embracing a different culture, communicating with people who speak a different language, and practising back-to-basics medicine.

A dream to live and work overseas can become a reality with some planning. There are many resources and support available to help you plan and prepare for a journey of a lifetime. Knowing where to start the process, narrowing down your choices and making key decisions well in advance can be beneficial in securing your ideal placement.

Developing good relationships with your supervisors, asking questions and volunteering to help wherever you can will enable you to build their trust, gain rich learning experiences and get the most out of your elective.

There may be a shortage of medical supplies and the equipment can be inadequate; however, the professionalism and dedication of local staff is inspirational. I have gained a lot of respect for what the local doctors and nurses are able to achieve with such limited resources.

As the doctors of tomorrow, you are helping to make an impact by improving access to health care for everyone – globally – so feel proud about deciding to do your medical elective overseas, and have an awesome time.

ADDITIONAL INFORMATION

I encourage medical students to embark on the journey of a lifetime during their medical elective and hope that you now feel equipped to plan your placement and get the most out of it.
If you would like more advice or assistance, please get in touch.

Contact me through our website: **www.doctours.com.au**
There is additional information and plenty of resources available on the website.

We are also on social media and you can contact us via:
Facebook: **www.facebook.com/doctoursvolunteers**
Or you can email me at: **karin@doctours.com.au**

CPSIA information can be obtained
at www.ICGtesting.com
Printed in the USA
BVHW091123140619
551042BV00022B/978/P